The User

Aidan Macfarlane is the Director of the National
Adolescent and Student Health Unit in Oxford. He is a Consultant in
Public Health Medicine, a Consultant Community Paediatrician and
an Honorary Senior Clinical Lecturer in Paediatrics at Oxford
University. He has co-authored a number of books with Dr Ann
McPherson, including *The Diary of a Teenage Health Freak*, *I'm a Health
Freak Too!*, *Me and My Mates*, *The Virgin Now Boarding* and, most recently,
Fresher Pressure. His unit advises NHS Commissioners on adolescent
behaviour and is involved in a number of national and international
research projects concerned with adolescent and student health.

Magnus Macfarlane is 24 and has degrees in Sociology
and Overseas Development. He has extensive first-hand knowledge of
illegal drug taking in young people having been involved with a
major thesis on 'The Culture of the Rave Scene'. He carried out most
of the interviews in this book through his contacts in the drug-taking
scene. After working at the Environmental Change Unit at Oxford
University and for Oxfam, he is now doing a doctorate in 'Social
Impact Assessment' at Bath University.

Philip Robson worked as a hospital doctor and clinical
pharmacologist before training as a psychiatrist. Having worked in
drug dependency units in Melbourne and London he developed a service for drug users in Oxford. He is currently a Consultant
Psychiatrist and Senior Clinical Lecturer at the University of Oxford.
He has published numerous articles and papers on drugs and related
issues, and, more recently, a book on the subject: *Forbidden Drugs:
Understanding Drugs and Why People Take Them*.

The User

The truth about drugs,

what they do,

how they feel,

and why people take them

Aidan Macfarlane

Magnus Macfarlane

Philip Robson

Oxford New York

Oxford University Press

1996

Oxford University Press, Walton Street, Oxford OX2 6DP

Oxford New York
Athens Auckland Bangkok Bombay
Calcutta Cape Town Dar es Salaam Delhi
Florence Hong Kong Istanbul Karachi
Kuala Lumpur Madras Madrid Melbourne
Mexico City Nairobi Paris Singapore
Taipei Tokyo Toronto

and associated companies in
Berlin Ibadan

Oxford is a trade mark of Oxford University Press

First published 1996 as an Oxford University Press paperback

British Library Cataloguing in Publication Data
Data available

Library of Congress Cataloging in Publication Data
Data available

ISBN 0-19-286179-4

10 9 8 7 6 5 4 3 2 1

Designed and typeset in Swift and Meta by Phil Baines
Printed in Great Britain by Mackays of Chatham PLC
Chatham, Kent

This book is dedicated to the affectionate memory of Jonty Ledger who was, before his tragic death, going to help to carry out the main part of the background research for this book.

Acknowledgements

We are extremely grateful to all those who agreed to be interviewed. All the interviews, which were tape recorded, are genuine but because of the sensitive nature of the subjects covered all the names have been changed to protect the confidentiality of those who agreed to be interviewed, except for Chief Inspector Andy Smith and Dr Philip Robson.

'The Facts' have been gleaned from a wide variety of sources which are listed under 'Further Reading' on page 152. We are extremely grateful to those providing this information.

Special thanks also to Ann McPherson and Ann Klaus for their support and their helpful comments and suggestions, and to all those who work alongside AM for their patience, humour and comments—Fiona, Ros, Julia, and Susanna; and to Becky for all her support to MM.

We are very grateful to Nick Blinco for permission to publish the interview with 'Ben', which was recorded as part of his thesis on 'The Social Context of Ecstasy Used in a College Situation'; also to John Balding for permission to quote material from *Young People in 1995*.

Finally a continuing thank you to Marny Leech who did the copy editing, for her care, patience and understanding. The reassurance of having her work on a book is inestimable.

Contents

Glossary

acid	LSD or lysergic acid
amyl	amyl nitrite
angel dust	phencyclidine (PCP)
bingeing	prolonged bouts of using cocaine or crack
blims	small fragments of cannabis resin
blow	cannabis
blowback	occurs between two people, one inhaling the spliff, the other inserting the burning end into his/her mouth and blowing back the smoke into the other's lungs
bong	large pipe for the quick inhalation of cannabis
bosh	to consume a drug
brown	heroin
bucket bong	a device for the quick inhalation of a heavy dose of cannabis which combines a bucket of water and a plastic bottle
buzzing	being high on drugs
busted	caught with drugs by the police
caned	high on drugs
carped	high on drugs
Charlie	cocaine
chilled out	relaxed
chillum	small pipe for smoking cannabis
chippers	occasional heroin users
clucking	withdrawing from any drug
coke	cocaine
crack	a form of cocaine that is short acting and highly addictive
cut	mix drugs with other substances
dope	generally cannabis but may refer to other drugs

downers	sedative type drugs
draw	cannabis
E	ecstasy
eggs	Temazepam
flashback	a reappearance of sensations associated with acid taking when not actually on acid
gauched out	extreme sedation on drugs
GBH	from GHB, a drug called gammahydroxybutyrate
grass	cannabis
hash	a form of cannabis
hot rocks	the burning blims from cannabis resin
House	form of dance music associated with the rave scene and ecstasy use in the late 80s and the 90s
huffing	inhaling solvents
ice	amphetamine
J	a joint
jellies	Temazepam
Jungle	type of dance music with a very rapid beat
kak	impure
lick the rock	take crack
line	powdered or crushed drugs snorted through the nose
monged	'out of it' when on drugs
microdot	small drop of dried lysergic acid on a piece of blotting paper
munchies	sensation of hunger after using cannabis
nicked	arrested by the police
ninebar	nine ounces of cannabis
'off it'	'out of it'
oil	class 'A' extract of cannabis, highly potent
para	paranoid
PCP	phencyclidine
pebbles	crack
pigs	police
poppers	amyl nitrite
pot	cannabis

puffing	smoking cannabis
reefer	joint
Rizla	make of cigarette papers commonly used for rolling spliffs
roach	rolled card inserted into the end of a spliff to make the draw easier
rock	crack
rush	an exhilarating physical high usually in the context of ecstasy use
score	buy drugs
scud	crack
skin up	make up a spliff
skunk	powerful hybrid cannabis plant
snidey up	mix the real ingredient of illegal drugs with other substances
snorting	sniffing drugs
speed	amphetamine
spike	add a drug to what someone is taking without their knowledge
spliff	joint of cannabis
squeeze	a good deal on anything including drugs
stacking	taking drugs in the right mixtures and with the right timing to get maximum effect
stepping on	mixing drugs with other substances
Techno	dance music with a repetitive beat: an up-tempo and more aggressive form of House
tolerance	needing to take more and more drugs (or drink) for them to have the same effect
toot	heroin
tranx	tranquillizers
trip	prolonged high from acid or mushrooms
uppers	amphetamine
valis	Valium
weed	cannabis
whizz	amphetamine
wraps	powder-based drugs in small hand-made envelopes containing one gram amounts

Rachel is a user.

She is 16 and studying for her A levels at a North London school. Her father is a doctor and her mother works in an advertising agency. After university she wants to make documentary films.

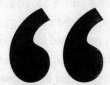

The first time I tried drugs was when I was about 11. I was on holiday in Wales with a group of mates who were all older than me—most of them were about 15 I reckon. I liked it—it was kind of cool, if y'know what I mean. It was fitting in that mattered. I mean, after being a kid I enjoyed it. I puffed before I smoked any fags. I never smoked fags much till now. I always stopped and started. I was never a real fag person.

I did mushrooms after that, on another holiday. I was about 13. My mate Chrissy and me went down to the beach. We didn't know anything about mushrooms. We didn't know how to take them, what they did to you, anything. We didn't have a clue. It was half term, and after taking them once, we took them the whole week. We thought they were wicked. We must have taken them four or five times.

Taking drugs blatantly changes you—it puts a new perspective on life. You see things differently. For a while I thought they made you a bit more perceptive—about stuff like relationships. Also, with trips on acid, you can find something interesting about the most boring things. That's a major attraction. You don't actually have to do anything exciting when you're tripping—it's just all there.

It's a bit like being born again. It takes you back to when you're a little child, all innocent, just sitting there, finger in your mouth, looking like a geek.

Interestingly, doping up for me has always been with older people, because I started earlier than my same-aged friends. So age doesn't really make any difference, apart from the 40-plus year-olds who seem a bit weird. I think that everyone I know who is like above 40, and is puffing, is actually quite mad. I really do. But then most people over 40 have lost it anyway. When I'm an old fogey, I'm going to live outrageously in Amsterdam, but in the in-between bit, I can see myself stopping—when I start doing more interesting things.

At my age, you spend so much time just sitting around with your mates not really doing much. You don't have that many interests, so there's nothing to stop you puffing. Puffing allows you to be bored.

All my friends puff—everyone, but that's just the way it's gone, because I've been puffing every day for a while now. I'm sure that when I started all my friends didn't puff, but now, even though I didn't notice it at the time, I've phased out the ones that don't. That's the way it goes. I think partly the reason for that is because people who don't puff hate it. I mean, they're just sitting there watching you doing something which for them is utterly boring. They're not caned, so they're just spectators at something they can't actually visualize. People who don't puff are on a completely 'other' wavelength and never get off their face.

Drugs and the music scene isn't so specially linked now—though personally, I listen to a lot of different types of music. Two or three years ago no one would go out without doing an E—no one. But now the scene's changed. Think about it. Everyone is Junglist now, and if you go and take an E on Jungle stuff, you're going to have a downer, know what I mean? Also, in general, people are not dropping E so much when they go out—whatever they're going to.

You get people taking crack with Jungle—though I don't know anyone personally. No—hang on—yes I do. Mike Reeney, he and his friends do—but they're idiots. Our age group are more into Charlie now. If I was going to take an E, I would go out to Techno myself—but I don't go out all that much. I did go to a House party last week. There's not so much drug taking with House. It's a bit more laid back.

Recently, because I've been puffing so much, I've had no money to go out. I would love to, but come the end of the week, I'm skint. On Friday night, if it comes to going out or getting a draw, I get a draw. Three of us get a half every week, which lasts till Sunday lunch-time maybe, and if we have the cash we'll get more.

The music scene is quite clear. There's Jungle, and people still E with Jungle, but not the two or three Es that they used to. The trendy Whirly Gig people are completely into speed and Es. That's mainly in East London. Then there's Hip Hop, but I've never been to Hip Hop. I'd like to though.

It's all right being a girl going out in London, but I would hate to be a boy. It's all aggro with them. I'd be really scared, but being a girl, you don't run into that scene. There's a North/South scene in London though. If someone from the South finds you're from the North, they tell you to fuck off. The North/South divide is serious. They positively hate one another. That's how it is at the moment, but it'll change. It always has to be something though.

Recently we've been doing some trips—acid, anything, it just depends what's coming in. One of us came by some microdots, so that's what we've been doing. Our favourite drug is weed skunk. Skunk is wicked—it's so strong and not like normal weed. It gets you just right, and you can't go out because you'd never be enough on the ball. It's a totally other experience, definitely a great buzz—skunk. Virtually like tripping—kind of like boiling inside your head.

There was this day in Amsterdam we were doing skunk. We sat in a café from seven-thirty in the morning smoking it, and we had to go to bed at four in the afternoon because we couldn't last out and we were so out of it. Just complete indulgence. Four days in Amsterdam and we didn't go anywhere or see anything. I would've liked to have looked around, but I was too out of it. If I'd been there longer though, I probably would've calmed down on the puff side. I mean, we'd gone there for the education, but it turned out to be education of a different kind.

There have been periods when I've been really negative about puffing, but you can't get out of it. There's a gang of us who do it, and when you try to get away from it you can't. If you go and see these people, you're going to puff. It's a group thing—we keep each other going. If you don't want to puff, you can't go round there. That's the group of friends I've got.

It's not going to be like that for everyone. It's rather like having drinking partners, but it does stop you doing other things. Like today, me and Josie said, 'Let's walk by the canal,' but then said, 'What's the point? We don't have spliff to do the walk on—so let's not go for the walk.' There didn't seem to be any point.

There are so many things which are better when you are caned—like school. I mean, school is just a hundred times better caned. No, actually that's a load of bollocks. I don't go for that at all. I don't puff in school ever. You'd never get anywhere that way.

I've cut down on puffing a lot. I can not have a spliff one day and now really not worry about it. It wasn't always like that. It used to be that I would start biting my nails if I didn't get a spliff. Stupid—it was plainly psychological. Now I just don't wind myself up so much about it. If I could only have one drug of all of them it would be weed.

Sex and enhancing drugs is a scene. I know couples who do Es who can only get off when they're on them. So many people are like that and can only have good sex if they're on E. Then they're at it like rabbits. It doesn't turn me on though—I mean, having to score drugs every time you have sex. That would be ridiculous, more hassle than it was worth. Not to get on unless you're on something— that's really sad.

I find what the government says and what parents say about drugs is bullshit. 'Don't take these drugs, they're illegal. They'll lead on to harder drugs. If you take acid, you'll see these 3D hallucinations for ever after.' I think that as soon as someone tries drugs and finds it's not like that and finds the pluses, they try doing it again.

You know the way they always say that soft drugs lead on to harder drugs, well that pisses me off. I mean, I understand what they're talking about. It does lead on to stronger drugs because you get a buzz on one drug which leads on to the need for a stronger buzz. Once you get a taste for buzzing, those buzz cells just have to be fed. It starts off an appetite for it, which has to be satisfied. But I think if you're going to do hard drugs, you're going to do them whether you're puffing or not—d'you know what I mean?

Drugs are a definite escape—from boring normality.

They've also got something to do with going against society. It's another one of the little things you're going to do so that you're not like everyone else. Every drug I take seems to show me a new side to my personality. It's not just an escape—it's an enhancement as well. But it's also a bit of a rebellion, at our age, against parents.

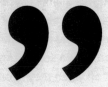

Facts:
Drug taking in general

The most commonly used drugs are

Caffeine   Used by both young and old in tea, coffee
and soft drinks. Although it does alter mood to a mild
extent, there is no evidence that caffeine alters people's
behaviour to any great degree.

Alcohol   The second most commonly used drug
by young people, and the second most dangerous drug in
terms of the number of deaths it causes. These deaths are
the result of alcohol's immediate effects in altering perception (especially where road traffic accidents are concerned)
and its long-term physical effects. Alcohol does change
people's behaviour even after only relatively small
amounts.

Tobacco   The third most commonly used drug by
young people. By the age of 16:

●   one-third of young people will have tried
smoking and will continue

- one-third will have tried and given it up
- one-third will not have tried.

Like caffeine, tobacco does not change people's immediate behaviour to a significant degree, but tobacco is by far the most dangerous drug in terms of killing people in the long run. If you give up smoking before the age of 24 (hard to do owing to the hugely addictive nature of tobacco), there will be no long-term effects. Giving up at any stage is beneficial.

Cannabis   The commonest *illegal* drug, with a
million plus regular users in the UK, followed by amphetamines and the other 'hard' drugs. The long-term health effects of smoking cannabis, as far as the risk of developing lung cancer is concerned, are at least as dangerous as smoking tobacco.

Total deaths from illegal drugs in England and Wales are about 1,200 per year. Total deaths from alcohol are about 60,000 per year. Total deaths from smoking cigarettes are about 110,000 per year. However, these number of deaths are relative to the number of people actually using drugs, alcohol and cigarettes, and for how long they use them. For example the deaths due to cigarettes are in people who have smoked for years and years, whereas significant illegal drug use is really only in people between the ages of 16 and 24.

Many people believe that if you start taking cannabis, you will almost always go on to taking harder drugs. Is this the truth or a myth? The answer is:

- if there is a tendency to progress from one drug to another, it starts with the caffeine in tea, coffee and Coca Cola, goes on to alcohol and smoking, then on to solvents, cannabis, amphetamines, cocaine and heroin

● young people may stop anywhere along this route. Only about 40 per cent of those drinking tea and coffee are going to go on to using cannabis, and only a minute number of cannabis users (less than 5 per cent) are going to go on to trying heroin

● what leads someone to start taking stronger and stronger drugs is not so much the drugs themselves as the personality of the user and their social, mental and physical circumstances

● cannabis, unless taken regularly in large quantities, is not addictive

● cigarettes are said to be as addictive as heroin

● exposure to the 'soft' end of drug taking is likely to expose you to people dealing in, and using, the harder drugs, thus increasing their availability.

All this suggests that in some ways legal drugs might do more damage than illegal ones, so why is there so much fear about illegal drugs?

● people are not sufficiently well informed about their effects, both pleasurable and dangerous

● there is a relatively small but definite health risk to drug taking. The deaths associated with the use of illegal drugs are usually well publicized on television, radio and in the newspapers because they have a 'sensational' aspect

● some drugs make people behave irrationally. We fear irrationality because it can harm the individual taking the drug, and because he or she may harm those nearby

● reality is hard enough to cope with, without the use of mood-altering drugs. These drugs often make matters worse rather than better when taken in an uncontrolled way

● illegal drugs are often impure or contaminated

● the illegality of drugs makes their price artificially high, making an addiction, particularly to the harder drugs, appallingly expensive. The huge profits involved lead to crime and violence, so the market rather than the drugs themselves has become something to be feared

● the illegality of drugs means running the risk of involvement with the police. This can lead to disturbing experiences with lifelong effects

● one of these effects is that you might have difficulty getting a visa for visiting other countries.

Jan has never used drugs.

She is 16 and training as a dancer at a London dance school. She has two brothers and her family live in Peckham where she attended a local state school. Her parents know nothing about her brothers' drug habits.

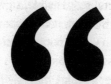

So why the hell have I never tried drugs—never at all? I've been offered them sometimes. They've not exactly been pushed at me, but they've certainly been available. I've a couple of girlfriends who are heavily into dope, and they occasionally say 'Do you want a puff?' but it doesn't interest me. I even know the occasional person who gets coked up when they go on stage. It's a way of giving them-selves nervous energy and getting over any stage fright—whatever; and stops them getting off by eating. Some of them are amazingly skinny.

What's put me off drugs is my cousin Dan who OD'd and died on heroin last year when I was about 15—he was 18. He'd started on dope and stuff, and had got himself into this state where it was totally uncontrollable, and this did me in for drugs. From what I've heard, he had this bag of heroin in his room and heard these police sirens. He thought they were on their way to get him, didn't he? There was this knocking on the door of his room and he was convinced it was the heavy brigade (when do they ever knock?) so he swallowed the whole lot. It was actually just his friends and a totally unlucky accident that they appeared just after a police car with a siren had gone by.

They got him to hospital as fast as they could but he died anyway. My mother told me all this and it freaks me out that someone could get themselves into a state where their minds are not working rationally.

Me, I think you've got to be responsible for your actions, and if you get to the point where you're not, then you've got problems. We've all got to the stage where we were really drunk and were not responsible, so we can't claim we don't know what it's about. It does show what you're capable of doing when you're out of control though.

I mean, drinking is easier to control, isn't it? You can have more of it with less effect. I think that having one joint is the equivalent of, say, six drinks, but I don't know whether that's a true estimate because I've never smoked. With drinking you can feel yourself getting out of control and you can do something about it. Whether you want to or not is a different matter. When you have a joint, I imagine you have to wait a bit and then there is nothing you can do to stop the effects. That's how I see it.

These girlfriends—they're lighting up every day. I go round there on Sundays at midday and they'll just be getting up and lighting their first joint. By tea-time they're sitting there not capable of doing anything, and they get so paranoid. They hear police sirens and go out of their minds. 'Quick, Jan, hide the stuff for us', and I have to bury it under plants and things. Seeing them in that state totally puts me off—it's just so gross. I don't envy their state of mind at all.

It's not as if I don't have any other contact with the stuff. One of my brothers, Ray, just takes dope and I hope it's something he'll grow out of. My older brother, Kev, does ecstasy and it makes me mad. It's just bloody stupid.

Last New Year I went out with him and a group of his mates to celebrate in a disco, and we ended up in casualty at Kings College Hospital. We waited there for four hours without seeing a doctor. Kev had collapsed a couple of times on the pavement outside the club before we went in, which really annoyed me. Then when we were inside and he'd had some more to drink, he had some kind of a fit and started thrashing around. The club had a paramedic who helped, but when the ambulance turned up the men in it instantly labelled him as drunk, or out of his mind on drugs. They didn't want to take him at first, did they? Just told us to call the police and were about to fuck off, but finally they gave in.

The doctor at the hospital, when he finally saw Kev, said it was a typical reaction that some people get to Es. Personally I had no sympathy for Kev whatsoever. I thought it was completely mindless to get into such a state. Everyone else was saying 'Oh, poor thing' and acting concerned. I was just mad as hell at him. What a stupid git to actually pay someone to do that to him. I mean, why?

I appreciate that us guys, at our age, need some kind of escape in our lives, but surely there must be other things to do? My own personal bag is meditation—no, don't laugh. Why not? I probably get just as high on that as other people get on dope. I mean, I do think that people need something to take them out of their mundane existence sometimes. I just don't think drugs are the answer.

Exercise and activity are another thing for me, definitely. I have to get my boyfriend to come and take me out for a walk—yes, just like a dog! It makes me happy, even if I've just finished dancing. Sometimes I have just too much energy.

I think I must be different from a lot of others, because apart from learning about my cousin I didn't really come across drugs until I met my two girlfriends. The thing with my cousin really scared me, and that was when I decided I would never get caught in that scene. It all seemed so foreign to me. When my friends started doing drugs, at first I was pretty frightened because I thought I might get sucked in. Then I gradually saw that it wasn't so very big deal. Occasionally I suppose they think I'm a bit of a killjoy, but they don't put on any pressure. They pass a joint around and say, 'Have a puff if you want to', but I never do.

As for why some people do drugs and others don't, I don't really know why. A lot of people say that you're a stronger person if you don't do drugs, but I'm not sure that's got anything to do with it. I know that my younger brother, who's 15, does it because it's relaxing. He's also into all this cool thing about fitting in with his mates—but I don't see him as a 'peer group pressure' victim. He enjoys it, and I think for him it's also the experimentation thing.

I smoked fags for two weeks just to try them, but I never really intended to take it up. Smelling other people's smoke is revolting enough. I played around with the image of it a little, sort of waved unlit fags around like some film actress. A friend of mine lit one for me once when I wasn't looking and I took a huge puff and nearly passed out. It was not nice of her, the slag.

I'm the sort of person who wears a cycle helmet and a safety belt. It just makes good sense to me. It's the same with sex. I would always make sure the bloke took precautions. No way would I sleep with anyone unless they used a condom. I'm not one for sleeping around. On the other hand, I'm not someone who puts absolute barriers up and says, 'No, I will never do that', because instantly it becomes taboo and then you want to try it, don't you?

Yes—I'm a vegetarian too, which may make me look like some sort of a health freak, but actually I'm a veggy because my family were too poor to afford meat for a time, so I just got used to not eating it. It's no big deal. I just got out of the habit.

My parents are blind naïve about the drug scene. I've been trying to make my mum more streetwise but they just don't seem to get it. I mean, I don't want to grass on my brothers, but they've got to be a bit more real. Drugs are much more normal now than when they were young. No way would they ever have been into that scene. Mum is terrified of even the word 'DRUGS'—it's really got to her that anything to do with drugs means instant addiction, brain damage, hospitals, death—all stuff like that in massive fluorescent lights. It's what she reads in the papers. I don't think Dad ever thinks about it, unless he discusses it with his mates at the pub. But he'd make a complete knockdown scene if he discovered what his kids are up to. I think it's wrong they should be like that because a 'shock, horror' scene is a total waste if you're going to be any help.

Kev thinks that if my parents did know about him and the Es they'd chuck him out, but they wouldn't, not at all. They're not like that when it comes to it. Yes, they're scared of drugs, but it's still family, isn't it? They'd be supportive. But he's reached the age when he's got to decide for himself, hasn't he?

Maybe people get into drugs because they can't see the good things in life and just want to escape. I'm not that negative type myself, and don't blame other people or drugs when things go wrong. At 15 it's also part of trying to sort out who you are and, like Kev and Ray, wanting to experiment with different attitudes and images. For myself, I think I have too much respect for my body.

The only time I was scared about drugs was when I read this story about a girl in America who was given an injection of crack in a shopping mall. Someone just put a needle through her jeans and loaded her with the stuff. That terrified me and I wouldn't go out on the street for a couple of days. But there's no real pressure on me. When it comes down to it, what can people do? They can't force the stuff on you.

It does worry me though that once you've tried dope you get the label of being 'a druggy' and people imagine you're in with a group of mates who are trying to persuade you to take harder stuff. I suppose addiction actually starts with tea and coffee, and then goes on to drink and fags, but to me those things are more controllable. I've seen people who have smoked a joint one evening and been totally unfit next day. All their energy and motivation seemed to have leaked away.

I think I've got my own addictions though—like exercise. I have this fixation about needing to move my body. If I had the cash, I'd spend it on working out every day. Steve reckons my addiction is shopping. Work is not an addiction because it's not important enough—not for me anyhow. What I enjoy most is my relationships—with family, with friends and with myself. I'm never bored. I just think up things to do.

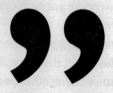

Facts:

Users and non-users of illegal drugs

How many young people take illegal drugs?

Different surveys give slightly different results, but all indicate that:

- ... by the age of 13, about 10 in every 100 young people in the UK will be offered an illegal drug
- ... by the age of 13, about 6 in every 100 will take an illegal drug
- ... by the age of 16, 50 out of every 100 will be offered an illegal drug
- ... by the age of 16, 30 out of every 100 will take an illegal drug (a total of about 210,000 16-year-olds)
- ... up to the age of 20, the absolute numbers increase but the proportion of those being offered drugs who actually take them remains much the same—that is, just over half
- ... the age of maximum drug use (in terms of the number of people taking them) is around 18 to 20: it then falls off rapidly

- • • drug taking among young people is rapidly increasing
- • • teenagers are starting to take illegal drugs at a younger and younger age
- • • the number of 15–16-year-olds trying illegal drugs has nearly tripled over the last 10 years
- • • the gap between what young people know about drugs and what their parents know is increasing
- • • the gap between what young people know about existing drugs and what they know about the newer drugs is also increasing
- • • although overall there is no difference in the extent of drug taking between young people who are well off and those who are poor, *compulsive* drug taking is more common among those who are living in poverty or are disadvantaged in other ways.

Why take drugs?

People use drugs because:

- • • they enjoy the effects
- • • drugs get rid of feelings of shyness, anxiety, and lack of confidence
- • • their friends are doing it and they don't want to be different
- • • taking drugs makes them feel rebellious and individual
- • • they will try anything once, out of curiosity
- • • drugs make poverty, depression, abuse more bearable
- • • the sensations they offer are better than boredom.

The reason may be any one of these factors, but is more likely to be a combination of several. When young people themselves have been questioned:

- ... 50 per cent say they take drugs for fun and/or out of curiosity
- ... 30 per cent say their friends are all doing it
- ... 20 per cent say it is a better alternative to worrying about something in their lives, or it makes them less anxious.

There are three main types of illegal drug users:

- ... by far the largest group of young illegal drug users are the experimenters (see Rachel, Simon and Robert) who try, say, cannabis (the most commonly used drug in the UK) a couple of times, enjoy it, but then abandon it for some other new experience (like sex, travel, or drink).
- ... the second most common group, also widely represented throughout this book, are the social users (see Guy, Ben, and John) who take drugs in the same way that they might go down to the local pub for a drink: something you do with friends, on a moderately regular basis.
- ... the third, and by far the smallest group, are the serious or 'compulsive' drug users, or 'addicts' (see Ian and Sara). In this group, drug taking may well be a symptom of other problems: severe socio-economic circumstances, a back-ground of abuse, unhappiness, and so on.

Some general points about illegal drug users:

- ... most drug users experiment with small quantities of drugs, infrequently, for brief periods
- ... therefore most people using illegal drugs neither seek nor need help
- ... and most people who use drugs socially never come into contact with the medical services, the police, drug counsellors, or anyone else concerned with illegal drug use.

However, illegal drug use is higher:

- ... in young people from single parent families
- ... where there is conflict within a family
- ... in families where there is already someone into illegal drug use.

Drug users who develop drug-related problems have lower self-esteem than non-drug users, but this is as likely to be the cause of drug taking rather than the effect.

The experimenters tend to be people who like to experiment in general, and therefore they:

- ... have an increased liking for alcohol
- ... are more likely to smoke
- ... are less likely to wear cycle helmets and seat belts
- ... are more likely to have started having sex earlier and to have more sexual partners.

Experimentation does not, however, appear to vary in any particular social group, rich or poor.

Why has there been a recent increase in the use of drugs, world wide and in the UK?

Drugs are much more easily available nowadays, and there has been an increase in the variety of drugs: uppers, downers, those that give you hallucinations, those that heighten sexual arousal. There is a growing menu of drugs for every occasion.

The availability and the variety have both developed because there is money to be made from drugs. The creation of a new drug with even better effects than the old one (crack being developed from cocaine, for example) means that dealers can sell more, and at a higher price.

Sammy is 13 and in her last year at the local

middle school. She lives with her mother, Dorothy, and her grandmother on a housing estate on the edge of Birmingham. She has a younger brother aged 10.

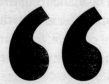

I think the thing with drugs is getting quite bad because there are so many people doing it. And the people that are dealing in it, they get into groups or gangs and pressurize people. I learn about these things from reading the newspaper or seeing about them on telly or in the magazines I read. *Mizz* and *Just Seventeen* have articles in them about how kids have been given something at a rave party, and they didn't know what was in it, and they ended up in hospital.

I think you can have your fun without taking drugs. Most people take them because they're pressurized. And there are people taking them in front of their mates to impress them, and when they're out — to have fun.

I think that they shouldn't take them because it can damage their health, and maybe they could die from them if they take too many. But that depends on how long they take them for. If they try once, then I don't think they will suffer any damage. From what I've seen on telly, it's when they take them all the time, at discos and things, that they end up in hospital.

Smoking ordinary cigarettes is stupid too. I tried one once. I was kind of slightly drunk at a party with my mum and she didn't know and someone put one into my hand. I took one puff and it didn't have any effect or anything—like feeling sick—but that was the only time. Mum is really strict about things and I like that. The only time we have a drink is when it's like a birthday party or something.

The drugs I've heard of are dope, speed, wacky, coke. I know a few people at school who are taking drugs, but it's not common knowledge and only a few people know who they are. I don't know anyone who is dealing with drugs in school.

My mum doesn't like anything to do with drugs. She tells me that if anyone pressurizes me to take them, just to walk away, and not ever to take them, or I could end up in hospital and die.

I do know some people who take them and I think they're stupid. I know one girl who does it sometimes, but not regularly. She does it to impress the boys she hangs around with. It's a sort of gang who do drugs.

Nobody has ever offered me drugs though. It's not as if anyone at our school is saying, 'Come on—you've got to try this.' There really are only a few who take drugs at my school, who want to look hard and that. Most of my friends don't, but we're only 13.

At my next school it may be different, especially from 15 onwards. It's that kind of age that are mainly into drugs I think, but I don't know whether I would try them in the future. You just can't tell. There are no attractions that I can see.

There is a drug scene on the estate here. I know a few people around here who take them—because a friend of a friend of mine tells me what's going on. They seem to do it in groups, sort of meet up and have a quick smoke of something. I think I would recognize the smell of cannabis. You did get it on the bus sometimes in the past, but now smoking cigarettes has been banned. I don't find needles or anything like that, but then I'm not looking, am I? Drugs don't frighten me. It's just not something I would have anything to do with.

What I like to do is running and sprinting. And whenever I can, I get down to the leisure centre and go swimming or play games or something. I'm never bored. I'm thinking of being a PE teacher when I grow up. Running is my best thing—sprinting but not long distance—and javelin and badminton. I was in the school football team. I was mid-field.

"

Dorothy, Sammy's mother

"

I've talked to Sammy about drugs—especially with this new school she's going to go to, with them older kids. She knows what she should do. I'm very old fashioned when it comes to that scene. I know there were drugs in my time, but I never tried them myself because I knew what they did to you. I say to her, 'What kind of life do you want?' Does she want the kind of life where she might kill herself, or does she want the kind of life where she has her own home and her own family? But I can't always be there for her. She's got to have her own standards and respect herself, like I did.

I was brought up strictly myself. My mum brought us three children up by herself and we never got into trouble. I never got pregnant, or took drugs. Mum brought us up right and I never did that kind of thing. We've always been a close family even if we do have our ups and downs. But my mum always told us, 'Outside this door is a rough world, and it's your choice, what you want.' She told us about what drugs could do to us, even if it wasn't sort of advertised then.

But with Sammy, when we're on our own and out together, and we see these kids in town who look like they're on drugs, Sammy says to me, 'Mum, I don't want to end up like that,' and I say to her, 'Well, you don't have to end up like that. You're a responsible young lady, you know what's right and wrong.'

You read about drugs everywhere now. It's on telly and in the newspapers, and when I go down and visit the doctors, they have these notices all over their walls. There's a boy in Sammy's class (and she'll probably kill me for saying this), and his mother is on her own. All she cares about is going out to discos and she leaves her children in alone. The boy is Sammy's age and he has two older brothers. His mum doesn't know it, but when she's out of the house, there's drug smoking there. Now where's the mother? The way I am, I wouldn't leave my kids on their own like that.

I think the reason for drug taking going up is family break-up, money, and lack of jobs myself. There's no close-ness of the family any more, no one seems to sit with their families any more and read, like we do. All this week we've done things together. Maybe it's the pressure of life. I don't know.

Sammy and I, well, we discuss things. I don't tell her what to do. I trust Sammy and she knows I trust her. I've got respect for her and she knows it, and she's got respect for me too. It's not me just saying, 'No, you can't do that'—we talk about it. I'd trust Sammy with my life, she's like my right arm. I know she wouldn't do anything like take drugs.

As she gets older, all I can say to her is, 'It's a tough world out there, and I'm here if you need me.' I'm not going to say to her, 'Look, you've got to do this, or you've got to do that', but rather, 'You've got to make your own decisions.' I mean, we all make mistakes, don't we?

There is a drug scene here on the estate. There was a raid last week at the top of the road at four o'clock in the morning, with squad cars everywhere. Next morning we could hardly get out, with it all being sealed off. My kids know it's there, they've seen it. They know what it's about.

What I don't understand is the attitude, 'Let's get some drugs and have a good time.' I don't know why you can't have a good time without drugs myself. I mean, what do they do to you?—make you sick. From what I've heard, they can kill you. I just think it's silly.

There've been points in my life where I've thought, 'I can't take no more,' and I've thought, 'Where's the way out? Where can I go? What can I do?' I've known people who've taken drugs just to block everything out. Maybe I've been that close myself, but I have to be responsible for my kids. I brought them into this world. I'm not going to kill myself and let them go into homes. No way. They're mine, they're my life.

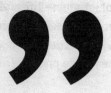

Facts:
The exposure to drugs

As young people grow up in the UK, exposure to news and information about the illegal drug scene is universal. It is virtually impossible for anyone to escape the coverage given to the subject on television, in newspapers, and in magazines.

Exposure to drugs is also first hand for large numbers of young people at school, in the community, and/or at work.

The Schools Health Education Questionnaire study, carried out by the Schools Health Education Unit at the University of Exeter, has looked at the life-style of thousands of children in the UK over the last fifteen years. The 1994 survey contains the following questions:

DO YOU KNOW ANYONE WHO YOU THINK TAKES ANY OF THESE DRUGS? [the drugs in question are: amphetamines, barbiturates, cannabis, ecstasy, cocaine, hallucinogens, heroin, crack, solvents, tranquillizers]

The percentage saying 'Yes' is given below, by the age of the children replying:

Age	Boys (%)	Girls (%)
11–12	14	13
12–13	30	32
13–14	46	49
14–15	63	67
15–16	71	73

So, at the age of 11 to 12, one in seven children think they know someone taking an illegal drug. By 13 to 14, this has risen to nearly half of the children, and by 15 to 16, nearly three-quarters.

A further question in the survey (to 15–16-year-olds) was: **HAS ANYONE EVER BEEN OFFERED, OR ENCOURAGED TO TRY, ANY OF THESE DRUGS?**

The percentage answering 'Yes' is shown below:

Drug	Boys (%)	Girls (%)
Amphetamines	18	18
Barbiturates	3	3
Cannabis	42	37
Ecstasy	14	15
Cocaine	3	3
Natural hallucinogens	15	11
Heroin	3	2
Crack	3	3
Solvents	11	11
Tranquillizers	3	3
Other illegal drug	3	3
None of the above	53	55

Cannabis has been, and remains, by far the most common drug both offered and used, followed by amphetamines, natural hallucinogens (magic mushrooms), and ecstasy.

These figures indicate how essential it is for parents to be informed about the drug scene in order to be able to educate children about drugs and how to handle being exposed to them.

If one in seven children aged 11 to 12 years is being exposed to drugs in his/her immediate environment, education about drugs needs to start then—if not before.

Simon occasionally smokes cannabis.

He is 16 and taking his GCSEs at a local state school in Leeds. His father is a relatively senior police officer and his mother, Liz, is a teacher. He has an elder brother, John, and a sister, Sara, both of whom are also occasional users of cannabis.

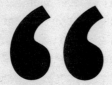

The first straight fag I had was when I was 11. I was given it by some 18-year-olds. I tried it, hated it, and gave it up. I smoked fags for six months when I was 13 and then I thought, 'Sod it, I'm not doing this any more.' Since then, I only smoke at parties and when I'm really stressed. Like most people, when I come out of exams, outside the school gates, where everyone has a packet, I immediately light up. You could create clouds in the sky with the amount of smoking that goes on there. But nobody I know actually puffs spliffs in school.

There's really no dealing in the school either. There are people at school I know I can go to, to get what I want. These people are right the way through all age groups, but they would never bring drugs to school. People know people, who know people, who know people and practically anything asked for can be got.

Virtually everyone is exposed to drugs, and I would guess that about half of my friends have tried cannabis. But most of them, like me, will have tried and then given up. It happens mostly at parties, when someone is handing around a joint and everyone takes a puff. It's almost exclusively grass, with the occasional odd mixtures. But sometimes something new comes along with a new mix of herbs—like there was something called 'cinnamon' recently.

It really is a party scene and unless you're a totally square sort of person, you're going to take a puff now and again. Occasionally someone offers something harder, but I've never tried any of that. That can mess your mind and put you out of control, and I've never been out of control—except when I've been drunk, but that's not the same. If you're drunk you do things and then wake up next morning and think, 'God, that was awful, what did I do?' but somehow you know about it. You might have no control, but you still know what's going on.

We've all done stuff that's really shameful when we were drunk. I know at least two girls who got so smashed they got into bed with the first person they've ever slept with and then felt rotten about it. Anyhow, cannabis, when you're high, is not a sexual turn on at all—it just lets you feel less worried about something or generally happier.

One thing I've noticed is that you either have heavy drinking parties or heavy puffing parties—or just a bit of both. If you puff, you don't drink heavily and if you drink heavily, you don't puff. If you're having a puffing party then it's just people having a good time. If it's a drinking party then things tend to happen.

The main reason for smoking cannabis at parties is that it's so bloody unsociable not to. You're talking away with a group of friends, and a spliff comes around and you puff. There's no pressure. If you passed it on, no one would call you chicken or anything, but it seems more natural to take a puff.

Also, it's fun—it makes it easier to talk to people and it's part of the scene. People have this thing about 'peer pressure', but I think that's absolute crap. It just doesn't happen. The reason one does it is because it's fun. It gives you a good time. If you're really bored with something—like for the last six months we've been working hard—after a while you just say to yourself, 'I'm sick of learning French verbs. I want to do something else.' You just want to lighten up a bit so you go off and have fun.

I don't think I'll get into trouble. The parties I go to are always with good friends and we look out for one another. Most of my friends wouldn't take more than grass anyway. Anything else can cause serious damage. You don't know what's in it and what it'll do to you. I don't want to see things which aren't there. With hard drugs, I'd be scared they'd get right inside my head.

I've never puffed in a public place, and it's never occurred to me that I might get arrested. If the police came round they might smell something at parties, but we deliberately don't make too much noise and stuff in case someone complains. It's usually music and talk. But the police wouldn't know who had been smoking. I mean, if I was the one holding the spliff, I'd get rid of it instantly, so how would they know?

I don't think my mum knows much about this or she wouldn't let me go out. She knows I've gone to parties and come back in the middle of the night smashed out of my head, because she's seen me. I expect she thinks I've probably tried grass. I get the feeling she thinks something is not right, but she gets the wrong idea quite often.

If she did know, I don't think she would go heavily overboard and ground me though. What she might do is give one of her awful 'Sit down and let's talk about it' lectures. I find them totally horrific, I'm not kidding. I don't want to be disrespectful here, but parents do go on a bit. We do listen to them, but it's like they're from another planet, the way they assume what we think. They're really weird that way.

Parents should say what they believe in though, and it must be very difficult for them. But if they go overboard and start yelling at you, you just switch off. Or you say, 'Right, well, if that's what you think, I'm not going to listen, and I'll not tell you anything from now on', in which case it's worse for both the parents and you—you because then you've got no safety net. If you're lucky, your parents will always be there if things go wrong. Mine would, I know— even with Dad's job which must give him cause to worry, I can see that.

You need your parents to know where you are in case something goes wrong, so I always tell them where I'm going. That's what parents are for, isn't it? To bail you out if the worst happens. The best line that parents can take is, 'Look, I don't want you to do this, and these are the reasons.' We need to be given limits, even if we don't always accept them. My parents certainly don't let me do everything I want to, and I respect them for that. It shows concern.

Another thing is, we know so much more about drugs than our parents do, unless they are into it too. I know one or two of my friends have parents who puff—not many though. This information we've picked up from our friends: what's the market, what people are doing, what the costs are, what the new names are, what happened to so and so when they took this or the other—stuff like that.

The main reasons for taking for me are: fun, not being unsociable at parties, availability, something you just do—like wearing clothes; not looking odd, trying it once as part of growing up. Most of my friends have tried it once—usually at a party—but that's all.

My advice to other kids would be: forget taking hard drugs because first, it will do for your mind, and second, it's incredibly expensive. Grass is easy and I've never known anyone seriously hooked on it. But hard drugs you get hooked on and you have to keep paying—with your health and your money. I'd never do hard drugs—under any circumstances whatsoever.

99

Liz, Simon's mother

66

I know that my children do take drugs—probably just cannabis, and probably out of curiosity or boredom. I don't actually know that Simon does. I know my oldest, John, has, and I would eat my hat if Sara hasn't. I haven't really talked to them about it because I think they don't feel confident that I and my husband won't disapprove, make a fuss, or be embarrassing about it. I don't think I would be like that, but it would probably depend on what sort of drugs it was. If Simon's smoking pot, I can't see what the fuss is about. I smoked it once myself, at a party, just before I became pregnant with John. It didn't do much for me. I've had no drugs before or since—it wouldn't be right with my husband's job and with me being a policeman's daughter as well.

Mine was a very protected upbringing. The one time I had the chance to try pot, I did, but it was just a one-off. I wasn't so impelled by curiosity that I was going to look for it and anyhow, I wouldn't have known where to begin. From 1962 to 1965, I was incarcerated in a totally female teacher training college, where you had to be in by ten o'clock. The warden would stand on the doorstep at two minutes past ten if you weren't there. You couldn't even go to a concert or a theatre. No sex, no drugs—they just weren't on the menu.

There was a patch after I left college and I was living in a flat in London when I can't think why I didn't take drugs. I suppose I just didn't come across that scene. So here I am, a policeman's daughter married to a policeman, and drugs are still beyond the range of my first-hand knowledge.

My attitude towards drugs for my children is that I can't say I worry about it. When Sara went to university I did worry a bit about things, including drugs. She's the one who's always been a bit subject to peer pressure and gets carried away. I did suspect she would hit the bottle hard, which she did, and I can see no good reason why she shouldn't have hit the drugs hard as well. Maybe she did, I just don't know. But in the same way as I think alcohol is totally evil when it's taken beyond moderation, I also worry about drugs beyond moderation, for the same reasons.

I never worry about Sara getting caught with drugs, maybe because I have this 'it will never happen to us' kind of attitude. I worry more about her health and what the effects might be of being really hooked on something which shifts your perception and the way you can work and be effective.

Sara is a bit extreme. She's either desperately miserable or desperately happy. I don't think she's desperately into drugs though. All that stuff about keeping an eye on your children, and if they seem gloomy or grey, whatever, might it be drugs? That doesn't occur to me, but I wouldn't really know what to look for. I wouldn't be into examining her arms for needle marks, or anything. It would be more a question of seeing how she reacts with me and other people.

Most of it is 'normal adolescence', isn't it? Complicated and unpredictable and emotional, and all the other things that make people say, 'If they are like this, maybe they are on drugs'. But that's rubbish—it's normal.

The other thing I worry about is the connection between normal experimentation with drugs and getting drawn into hard drug addiction. It's Sara I worry about most, but not really about drugs. I just worry about her generally, that's all.

John's different. He's very conservative, and would never take something if he didn't know where it came from. He wouldn't do anything that would seriously damage his health, or wreck his life chances. He's totally sensible.

Simon's different again. He's so well informed and so down to earth about the drug scene. I'd be surprised if he wasn't trying things out, but I think he's much more likely to say he's tried things out than actually to do it. He's a bit of a dramatist, but given the percentage of children who are trying drugs nowadays, it would be strange if he hadn't at least tried a puff of something. I can't remember exactly what the statistics are, but if I'm to believe Simon about his class then I would say that about half of them are on drugs, and nine out of ten of them have had sex.

If Simon has tried pot, I would want to know who is flogging it to them and what else they're being exposed to at school. Cannabis I could accept, but anything harder I'd want the authorities to know about. Simon knows about the effects and side-effects of drugs, and he knows what I think—though I've had such endless conversations about it all that I'm no longer sure what that is!

What I think he knows is that I know it's inevitable that sooner or later he will try pot, and I have no problems with that at all, even if I am a policeman's wife. I don't mind, provided he doesn't get hooked into some harder scene.

My concern as a teacher is that if there's a lot of smoking pot at his school, then it's likely to be among pupils who are working less rather than more, and I hope Simon doesn't get into that. It's not the drug taking itself that bothers me, but the life-style of those involved in it.

The trouble is that Simon feels that drugs is not a subject you discuss with your parents—and particularly with the ones he's got! Quite apart from having a dad who's a policeman, to him we're just 'Golden Oldies'. Things are changing though. There was a time when he would refuse to walk through town with us, and I was deeply embarrassed by my mother for much the same sort of reasons.

Incidentally, I do think that people who go on taking drugs after their early twenties are into something completely different from the experimenting of teenagers. For teenagers it's about being in the 'in crowd' and to do with uncertainty about the future. And crucial to all of it is availability—if you can't get drugs, you can't take them.

It sounds like an expanding menu though. If I had my life again, I'd probably be smoking pot like I drink alcohol now. I do have a horror of losing control—though to be honest, I don't mind being out of control if it's going to be nice.

If Simon, God help us all, did get picked up with drugs, I don't know how Jack, my husband, would take it. My first thought would be whether I should ring a solicitor or not. No, I think I would just rush down to the police station and worry about a solicitor later. If it was only cannabis, I would think that the law is ridiculous, and try to be open with the police and sympathetic to Simon—but I can see it would be awkward!

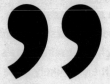

Facts: Cannabis

A 'Weed' Poem

Roll it, spark it, smoke it, love it,
    that's why the smokers stay;
    take a lug, feel the buzz, hear what the lyrics say.
Things are seen in a different light, waffle on all day;
    but going home to face your mum,
    you'll wish you'd stayed away.
You think she'll know, you know she'll know,
    your eyes are going red;
    you practise what you're going to say,
    round and round your head.
You stagger in, where's the switch?
    the stairs are never-ending;
    you reach the top, knackered and worn,
    Mum's stood there on the landing.
'Where have you been? What did you do?
    I've been worried off my head.
    You smell of smoke, you look like death . . .
    why are your eyes so red?'
Oh shit! When the para attacks
    it messes up my head.
    'Mum, I'll say "goodnight".
    I'm on my way to bed.'

(A regular user aged 17)

Cannabis is the most commonly used illegal drug. It is estimated that there are around 300 million recreational users in the world today, and between 5 and 10 million people in the UK have tried it at one time or another.

Its history

The taking of cannabis is nothing new. Its use as a medicine, derived from the hemp plant, was first recorded in Egypt in the sixteenth century BC and by the fourth century BC the Chinese were cultivating it. The Romans used the plant for rope-making and weaving, and brought cultivation to Britain where it became a major industry.

Although the use of cannabis to affect the mind was probably introduced into Europe about a thousand years ago, it did not become popular until the end of the nineteenth century—and then mainly among artists and intellectuals. Its full potential as a 'fun drug' in Britain was recognized in the 1950s when it was imported in quantity by Jamaican immigrants.

In spite of its medicinal effects as a painkiller, anti-convulsant, sleep inducer, and appetite stimulant, the use of cannabis was outlawed in Britain in 1928. Arguments about its legal status have continued ever since.

Large-scale scientific reviews have been carried out in several countries, including Britain, the United States and Canada. None of these has come up with evidence that occasional or moderate use of cannabis causes mental or physical illness, leads to antisocial behaviour, or alters the personality of users. In 1987, the British Royal College of Psychiatrists stated that ' . . . on any objective reckoning cannabis must get a cleaner bill of health than our legalized "recreational drugs".'

A synthetic cannabinoid called nabilone is being used legally to suppress some of the unpleasant side-effects of chemotherapy in the treatment of cancer; and the beneficial effects of cannabis are recognized by people suffering from other diseases, such as multiple sclerosis.

Its names

The formal names in the UK are marijuana and cannabis. Its street names are: BLOW, GRASS, WEED, HASH, POT, DOPE, SHIT, DRAW, WACKY-BACKY, GEAR, PUFF, and SPLIFF. In the East it has a number of other names: BHANG, CHARAS, GANJA, KIF, DAGGA, KABAK, and HASHISH.

Cannabis is usually mixed with tobacco, rolled into a cigarette, or 'joint', and smoked. The name 'joint' is now out of fashion, and has been replaced by 'spliff', 'bifter', 'cone' or 'two-skin'. When rolling a spliff ('skinning up'), the 'hash' is first 'toasted' and then put in rolling papers with tobacco and a 'roach'.

Its various forms

Cannabis comes from a plant known as cannabis sativa, which is a relative of the nettle and grows wild throughout the world. The plant is highly resinous, and a particularly potent form of dope, sinsemilla ('without seeds'), is obtained by culling the male plants before pollination occurs. This results in larger flowering heads in the female and abundant resin.

More than 400 chemicals have been found in the resin, including 60 compounds (cannabinoids) which have an effect on our perceptions. The most active ingredient is called delta-9-tetrahydrocannabinol (THC) and different forms of cannabis come with different THC levels (between 1 and 30 per cent THC by weight).

There are three main forms:

cannabis resin is a dark to light brown substance, scraped off the surface of the plant and pressed into a solid lump. It is usually mixed with tobacco and smoked.

marijuana and **grass** are the names given to the dried leaves and flowering tops of the plant. It looks like dried herbs and is smoked on its own or mixed with tobacco.

cannabis oil is a treacly liquid, refined from the resin or from the plant itself. It is smoked either mixed with tobacco or smeared on cigarette papers and rolled with tobacco.

New forms of the plant are being developed all the time around the world. Some of these are artificially engineered plants referred to as F1 hybrids. The strongest of these, developed in Holland, is currently held to be 'Northern Lights'. Other types include Purple Haze, Sumatran Red, Durban Poison and skunk.

'Blunts'—massive joints, the size of Havana cigars, are becoming very popular in the USA.

Although cannabis is usually smoked in the Western world, it is also effective if eaten.

Sources and cost

A huge amount of UK dope is home grown from seeds imported from Holland. Imported dope comes from Ghana, Nigeria, Jamaica, Morocco, Pakistan, Afghanistan and Holland. Lebanese and Nepalese hashish is now rare, as are 'Thai sticks'. The average price is around £25 for a quarter of an ounce of hash, which would make about twenty cannabis cigarettes. Home-grown dope tends to be cheaper and contains a lower amount of THC, though recently the amount of THC even in home-grown hash has become higher owing to better cultivation techniques. Cannabis is less adulterated than most drugs, but may be impregnated with hallucinogens such as PCP (phencyclidine) to increase its impact, and dope from Central America may contain toxic herbicides.

The effects

The average joint contains 300–400 milligrams of herbal material, but even the most expert smoker will not be able to absorb more than 1–30 milligrams of THC. The threshold level of THC that has an effect, however, is just 2 milligrams. The effects come on within a few minutes, peak after about 30 minutes, and last for 3–4 hours. If you eat the cannabis, onset is delayed for 1–2 hours, depending on when you last ate, and what you ate with it, but the effects last longer and their intensity is less predictable.

The effects of cannabis depend on your mood. Most users report that it brings on feelings of contentment, relaxation and happiness, that music sounds better, and everything around is enhanced. But cannabis tends to heighten whatever mood you were in before you took the drug, so depressed or anxious people may feel even worse.

On the physical side, you may become clumsy, your speech slurs and your eyes become reddened. Because cannabis reduces the ability to carry out complicated tasks, it should not be used if you need to concentrate on such activities as work, driving, or playing sport. It should not be taken with alcohol.

The bad effects

Fatal overdose from dope alone has never been reliably reported. Known side-effects, which are relatively rare considering how commonly the drug is used, include rapid heart beat, anxiety occasionally leading to panic attacks, and a degree of paranoia. Much less commonly, flashbacks, loss of mental control, and even madness have been reported. Of considerable concern, however, is the possibility of still unrecognised long-term effects, especially with the newer and stronger hybrids like skunk. If you suffer from psychological problems or have a bad trip using cannabis, you would be wise to avoid using it altogether.

One side-effect that gives serious cause for concern is the way the drug interferes with memory, in particular the ability to learn new information. Recent research suggests that this memory loss continues for several weeks after stopping using the drug. Cannabis certainly increases accident proneness.

Four spliffs a day are estimated to cause the same risks to the lungs as twenty cigarettes. However, while tobacco smoking is often a lifelong habit, very few people spend a lifetime smoking cannabis.

A passing concern for some males may be that THC seems to lower the sperm count, but luckily this appears to be a temporary effect. It is wise to avoid cannabis (and all other unnecessary drugs) when you are pregnant.

There is no evidence that cannabis is physically addictive, but it is possible to become psychologically dependent. Users come to rely on it as a way of feeling more relaxed socially. Abrupt withdrawal in heavy smokers may cause irritability and sleeplessness.

The law

The law hands out penalties up to a maximum of 5 years in prison for possession; and for supplying, an unlimited fine and up to 14 years in prison.

Robert was busted for possession of cannabis.

He is 16, is about to take his GCSEs at a local comprehensive, and has a sister, Janice, who is 19. His mother, Janet, who is interviewed here, works as a hairdresser in Nottingham and her husband is a manager.

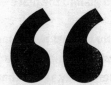

It was about midnight one Sunday. We had just gone to bed when there was this phone call to say that our son was sitting in a police station, having just been arrested for being in possession of cannabis.

I knew that both my kids had tried it. When Robert told me he had, we talked about it—the dangers of being caught with it basically. We talked about other people who smoked, and I warned him that it carried risks.

I never tried cannabis myself when I was young. What I knew about the drug was what I'd picked up by reading the papers and talking to some of my clients.

I didn't know enough about it and I've certainly learned a lot since, but not the way I would've wanted. I do know a lot of other kids who have smoked cannabis, and although I knew it was illegal and all that, it had attained a sort of degree of normality in my life. I just didn't think it would be one of my kids who got caught.

I thought my children were fairly sensible about what they do. They don't get drunk very often, and even when they do, they don't do it in public places. They are relatively law-abiding, I mean, they wouldn't go into a shop and steal things, or anything like that. In their minds, smoking cannabis just doesn't come into that category as I think smoking the stuff has got a general acceptance among teenagers.

What had happened in Robert's case is that a whole crowd of them—not the kids he usually hangs around with—had gone into a pub down in the town. They hadn't been drinking much, but only because they didn't have much money. Crowds of them go into the place—from their school and other schools.

I hadn't realized, but for the last twelve months or so Robert had been smoking cannabis fairly regularly. I don't think excessively—once a month, say, rather than weekly—with a crowd of friends, but in this case he wasn't with his usual group.

A crowd of them had been smoking—mostly sitting on a bench in one corner of the green where this pub is. None of them were smoking when the police arrived. A local resident had seen them and tipped off the police. They sent two police cars, three policemen, and two policewomen for a group of six kids.

They had jointly bought some cannabis from a dealer who was well known to all of them. Two of them, one being Robert, voluntarily gave some to the police. I mean, it was literally just a few strands, no more. The others had some which they swallowed. I suppose they were more streetwise than Robert.

Robert handed the stuff he had over to the police because they said to him, 'It will be much better for you if you give it to us. You'll probably just get off with a warning. We don't need to tell your parents, and you won't get into trouble.' These were all things which made him feel it was a better option, but they were very, very misleading. There was nothing about 'You'll have to come down to the station and give a statement,' and nothing about 'This will go down on your record' or 'You're under 17 and you need someone there before you give any statement.' They even said, 'Don't worry, we'll give you a lift home and your parents will never know.'

This made me feel absolutely furious. I mean, I was pretty cross with Robert, but I was far more cross with the police. He only had about six to eight strands of the stuff—a minute amount—and they said to me that normally, if they found kids with this amount, they'd just tip it down the drain and tell them not to be so stupid. They said that to me and to Robert. But they decided not to do that in this case because a resident had reported the teenagers. They felt they had to be seen to be taking stronger action.

Robert and the girl who had given the police cannabis were the only ones taken down to the police station and locked in cells. They let the others go. My first reaction when they phoned was, 'Oh God, well I suppose it's got to happen some day.' My second reaction was fury. Fury with Robert because he just hadn't thought things through, with him taking GCSEs and all that. And fury with having just gone to bed and having to get up again—the sort of normal parental fury at something happening over which I had no control.

We both went—me and my husband. It was a hassle and I was cross because Robert had been so stupid. Whether I was cross because I thought he was stupid for having taken the stuff in the first place, or because I thought he was stupid for having got caught, I don't know. I don't know if I can separate the two. It was the same kind of fury I used to feel if one of the kids got lost. I used to get frightened, and when I found them again, I was angry at them for having put me through it.

I went down and saw Robert in the cell and my husband stayed outside. I went into the cell and shouted at him, because frankly to find your child in a police cell is horrible. I know it was the wrong reaction, but I couldn't stop myself. I shouted at him for being so stupid and then he started to shake and I put my arms around him.

He absolutely did not weep. He just stood there and gave his statement, while all I could think of was whether the school would find out and whether he would be allowed to take his exams. I asked the policeman, 'What'll be the consequences as far as the school is concerned?' and he said, 'Well, we may, or may not, tell them.' I said, 'Please don't. He's just about to take his exams and they'll probably suspend him straight off.' But they wouldn't say what they would do and I hated them for that.

Robert was amazingly straight. He didn't panic and didn't say anything more than he needed to. He didn't mention his mates, or give names, or anything—nothing to implicate the others, though the police put incredible pressure on him. They also visited him at home a couple of days later and questioned him further when I wasn't present. Now I know more, I don't think they had the right to question him without me being there.

The statement was taken in the cautioning room and was tape recorded as well as written down. I reeled a bit under the formality of the whole thing. There were two police taking the statement, one a woman, both in uniform. They weren't unpleasant to Robert though. Then he was taken somewhere else and the senior officer said to him, 'You understand that this is a caution. We're giving you another chance, but if we see you again, you'll get a criminal record. This caution is also on file, and if you get caught doing anything else, wherever it is, it will be used against you. The caution will be on record until you are 17.'

I don't think it's sunk in with Robert yet—not fully anyhow. If anything, *anything*, happens again, he's going to have a criminal record. He's 16 now and this is going to hang over him for the next year. It's a long time.

We were in the police station for two and a half hours. We signed the statement and were on our way out when Robert said, 'Bloody hell, how can the police have such power? To ignore a tiny bit of cannabis and flush it away, or to decide to arrest you. It's totally amazing.' It seems amazing to me too.

But whatever Robert had thought about smoking cannabis before, there was no doubt in his mind now that it was illegal and that he had to accept the consequences. There was no way he was saying he shouldn't have been arrested—he knew the risks.

When we got home, we sat and talked about it. At first Robert denied having smoked on a regular basis, but then it came out that he had. My main feeling was, 'How could I have been so stupid not to have known anything about it.' Once you've got a criminal record, it's bloody awful and it's going to stick with you the rest of your life. It's always there against you and it damages your chances of getting jobs.

I keep asking myself, 'When did I take my eye off the ball? How could I have not noticed? Why did I trust him so much?' It's an impossible time, when they're saying, 'Trust me, let me get on with my life and be with my own friends.'

The good thing to come out of it is that we've had it all out, shouted a bit at one another and admitted that things have not been totally good over the last few months. My husband was a bit more detached about it all, though going to the police station and picking up his son was pretty awful for him. Afterwards he was more prepared to say, 'Well, what's been done has been done, so why don't we leave it at that?' But I think it probably went deeper with him.

I do think that my relationship with Robert had deteriorated a bit before all this happened, from something that had been extremely good and close to us going our separate ways with him needing his peers more than me. I mean, it's a period which has to be gone through, hasn't it? He had become socially orientated and just wanted to do what his friends were doing. I do worry about the future though, and it's hard to let go.

What have I learnt from all this? That parents need to realize that it can happen to *your* child. It's not always going to be someone else's, and not just what other people's kids do. And never believe what the police say because they're shits. They're used to dealing with low life, and even if you don't think your kids are low life, the police do. They treat everyone the same. The other thing is to find out much more about drugs, and why kids take them. The least we can do is be much better informed. Otherwise, how can we help?

And if you're going to warn your kids about drugs, saying 'You are not to do this' will have no effect at all. Instead, you need to say, 'OK, I know lots of kids are doing it and you'll probably come up against it yourself at some stage. We don't want you to do it, we'd far rather you didn't.

But if you do have to succumb to it, then for God's sake, do it in a totally private place—where people can't see you or get at you. And do it with people that you can trust absolutely—though that's easier said than done.'

I've warned Robert, 'You can't afford to do it again. Even if you're not doing it yourself but are just caught with someone else who is, you're very vulnerable and there will be some way in which you can be incriminated.'

One thing I was amazed about is how Janice, his sister, laid into him. Janice has experimented once, as far as we know, and she told us about it. But she was so angry about Robert putting his GCSEs at risk and upsetting the family, she slagged him off really hard. We're a close family and this really upset things, and Janice couldn't stand that.

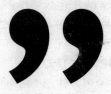

Facts:
If you get arrested

Each year in the UK, about 40,000 people get arrested for having illegal drugs on them. Drug laws are complicated. Do you know what is legal and illegal?

The Misuse of Drugs Act (1971)

The drugs covered by the Misuse of Drugs Act are:

CLASS A DRUGS: HEROIN, COCAINE and CRACK, LSD, ECSTASY, MAGIC MUSHROOMS (if made into a preparation), AMPHETAMINES (if injected).

Class B drugs: AMPHETAMINES and CANNABIS.

Class C drugs: weaker stimulants, most BENZODIAZAPINES and some other mild sedatives, pain killers and sleeping tablets.

The main offences
(in order of increasing seriousness) are:

* having small amounts of a drug for your own use
* having small amounts of a drug which you intend to sell or give to someone else

* having large amounts of a drug which you intend to sell or give to someone else.

It is also illegal:
* to grow or make these drugs
* to let someone use your house or flat to sell drugs
* to let someone use illegal drugs in your house
* to send drugs abroad, or have them sent to you.

The drugs which it is not illegal to have in your possession are: KETAMINE, POPPERS, STEROIDS, and TRANQUILLIZERS.

BUT, it is an offence under the Medicines Act for an individual to give or sell ketamine, steroids and tranquillizers to someone else.

Know your rights

The police have the power to stop people, search them, and arrest them if they think they are carrying illegal drugs. If this happens to you, you have certain basic rights:

* you have the right to remain silent and not answer any questions
* the police should have reasonable grounds for suspecting you and these should be explained
* if you are arrested, the police should explain what it is for
* the police should not take you to the police station unless they arrest you first, or you agree to go voluntarily

* if you are a girl, body searches can be carried out by women police officers only
* if you are under 17, the police should contact your parents or guardians and tell them why and where you are being held
* if you are under 17, the police should not question you without your parents or guardians being there
* you have the right to ask the police to notify a friend or relative if you are arrested
* if you are held in a police station or interviewed by the police, you are entitled to legal advice. If you have, or know, a solicitor ask if you may phone him or her. If not, ask for a solicitor under the Duty Solicitor Scheme, which provides one free of charge
* if you are arrested and taken to the police station, the police can hold you for up to 24 hours (36 hours for a serious offence) without charging you while they make further enquiries
* after that time, they should either let you go, charge you with an offence, or have a warrant from a court to hold you for longer without charging you.

Guy drinks and uses cannabis socially.

He is 20 and in his second year studying Economics at Edinburgh University, having taken a year off after leaving school to travel around the world. His father and mother run a pub.

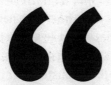

I think that the main reason people puff is out of boredom. Actually, the way I see it is that when you're born, everything around you must be new; and the first time you take a trip, everything is new and seen in a different light. Up to the age of 14 or 15, you're discovering things on a natural, normal level of thinking. So the mind gets used to seeing things in a new light all the time—a sort of natural instinct.

Also, particularly among boys, it has become a way of bonding, a sort of prop between them, which is perhaps why girls are less dependent on drugs. Although girls try drugs as much as boys do, they don't do it persistently over so long a time. Girls experiment, but want to stay in control more. For boys, it is the group thing that matters, and it is also a sort of 'rites of passage' thing.

I reckon my drug taking will fall off after the age of 22 or so, when I have to start thinking about getting a job and finding somewhere to live. Drug taking is not compatible with the mortgage life-style, if you like.

Drug taking at my time of life is an occupation in itself—especially if you're into dealing to fund your habit. Many people pay for drugs as automatically as they pay for food, in fact some that I know pay for drugs instead of paying for food. There's a real attraction there for some people.

I don't think families make any real difference as to whether we take drugs or not. I was talking recently to Jane, the mother of my friend Jake. She's a user, but she didn't smoke anywhere near Jake until he was 15. What happened then was, she was in the kitchen one day, cooking him some spuds, and he walked in with a spliff in his mouth. All this time she'd been hiding it away from him that she smoked, thinking perhaps that would keep him from taking it up. Maybe, in the end, it didn't have much relevance that his mum smoked. Or maybe they're just similar characters with the same kind of genes.

But there probably is an emotional reaction though. I think that if your parents are dead against drugs but don't know anything about them, it might make the attraction just that little bit greater—a bit of rebellion in fact. I also think that people from broken homes are more likely to be into drugs—to get away from all that scene. But it may be just to get away from harsh circumstances in general. It's another way of escape, isn't it? If you come from a more secure background, it mightn't stop you experimenting, but you might not need it so badly—the escape bit, that is.

So an element of it is escape, and an element is experimentation. I think when you're younger, it's more experimentation, but if it hangs on, then you're using it to try to get away from something else.

When you're on drugs, part of their beauty is that you're not living in the past or in the future. You live in the moment. You're not worried about what's going to happen tomorrow, you're not worried about what's happened in the past. You're living in the present, and that's what's terrific about it. I think that's why there's such a need for drugs now, because we're carrying this baggage of worries around—like unemployment. As soon as you decide to take a trip—a group of you, all mates together—that's it, the real world disappears.

The other beauty of it is, that if you take it as a group, you know that everyone is going to be there together for the next five hours. In this mad world, where everyone is rushing around and trying to change everything, here is a group of people who can do this one thing together and be on the same wavelength. It's a social thing for me—like going to the pub with my mates and having a drink. With some of my friends, like John, it's 'Let's go and have a pint,' while with others, Jake to name but one, it's 'Let's go and have a smoke.' It's just habit, I suppose.

Objectively, I have to admit that at some stage drugs can become antisocial. Over time, you stop talking when on drugs, and paranoia or neurosis can creep in. There's a neurotic side to smoking dope, which is why I now prefer drink. But then drink's just another drug. Drinking is definitely more sociable, though people need drink to sort of 'open up'. I think that some people start smoking because they hope it will help them to communicate, but it ends up making them communicate less.

Within the drug scene there are lots of subgroups—as there are in life in general, but if anything it's more intri-cate. There are groups that I drug with and groups that I drink with, and even other groups I drug and drink with. Certain people have a drinking mentality and certain people have a drug mentality, and some people can cross between the two.

I only occasionally smoked with my girlfriend—it's not the same as doing it with the boys. It's bonding with the boys, with your girlfriend, it's more of a laugh. Boys and girls don't communicate in the same way, which is what makes it difficult.

At school, I didn't know many girls who would go the full distance on drugs—getting completely mashed up and out of their brains. I think the motivation is the same— experimentation—but girls will stop at a much earlier stage. Also, they're much less likely to buy the stuff. Most of the time they'll get it off some boyfriend, or whoever.

Drugs are a boys' thing, even if the experimentation rates are similar. The people running it and dealing in it, and the people doing the most drugs, are boys. In addition to the bonding, there's the appeal of having a business to make money out of, and there's the drama side which people get a real rush from. Girls may try one spliff, or half an E or something, which will be enough for them, while their men will be getting completely off their faces.

How parents handle it is another aspect of it all. Parents need to say what they think, but let their children decide for themselves. They're not going to change what their kids do. They can't lock them up or whatever. The reality is that wherever a young person goes now, he's going to be offered drugs, so the idea of cutting out their availability is just not on. Parents need to provide what information they can, but it's got to be honest information not just the horrors.

My parents were very good—top marks, yes, top marks. I think I have a pretty balanced view of drugs thanks to them. It's not that they were too liberal or anything, just that they gave me the facts and let me decide. The facts and that it's illegal—that's what we need to know. Maybe children are not given enough credit for being able to decide for themselves if they are given the facts; but that shouldn't stop parents having opinions and expressing them.

I think the real question parents should be asking is why their kids need drugs in the first place. Beyond the experimentation is an emotional side which needs to be looked at. Take Jake for instance. I think for him drugs became a release. He always felt that people were down on him, and somehow the drugs scene got him round that as both user and dealer. I couldn't understand how someone like Jake could deal in drugs, because he objected to the whole money system by which dealing functions. It was a Catch 22 situation. He was trying to make enough money from drugs to get out of the whole scene, and then he goes and gets rumbled.

The whole business of dealing is self-destructive, particularly in Jake's case. There was this time when he came to Edinburgh and brought a kilo of gear with him. He was the usual shambles—didn't buy a train ticket, tried to dodge the guard, and arrived at an address he didn't know. He had to push the kilo through the door because there was no one in, and it wasn't even good weed. If it had been, it might have been worth it, but to run the risk of getting nicked for stuff that was unsmokable . . . . It was left there for three days with a note scrawled in crayon saying, 'Dropped this off, catch you later.' I mean, he was completely slack. When he got nicked, I was only surprised it wasn't earlier. No one is that stupid unless they want to get caught. Maybe in some perverse way he did.

Personally, for me now, I much prefer drink because it lets you stay in control. I think at some point you have to make a decision: which is more important—fantasy or reality. At the end of the day, you have to live in the real world and in the drug scene I know people who are totally out of it. I know, I've been there. At times I've been out of it for more than 50 per cent of the time. But the day will come when you say to yourself, 'I've got to get a job.' I don't know whether this is a choice you make, or a choice you are pushed into, but you do make it, and in order to do that you have to function on a normal level. Booze is much more amenable than drugs. It's more acceptable as well as being more controllable. This is not to say that you stop enjoying drugs altogether, it's just that you have to let go of them a bit.

When I was younger, I did try glue and Tipp-Ex fluid. I used to have it in class on my sleeve, sniff it and crack up laughing, but that didn't last long. It got around that inhaling things was dangerous. We all tried solvents, but none of us were serious 'gasheads'.

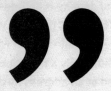

facts:
Inhalants/ solvents

Solvents are found in glues and adhesives, cleaning fluids, aerosols, petrol, rubber solution, correcting fluid, paint, varnish, nail polish, dyes, and room fresheners. Sniffing solvents is a cheap 'high' used mainly by children who can't afford alcohol and other expensive drugs.

A more sophisticated solvent is AMYL NITRITE, a liquid which, when inhaled, dilates the blood vessels, particularly those supplying blood to the heart muscles. It is legally prescribed for those suffering from angina and was popular in the 1960s, because as well as giving a short 'high', it was said to enhance sexual pleasure. It was sold off prescription in small gauze-covered glass ampoules which were known as 'poppers'. In 1969, amyl nitrite was made a 'prescription only' medicine and its popularity decreased.

BUTYL NITRITE and ISOBUTYL NITRITE are available in small bottles and are used legally to make rooms smell pleasant. Their effects, when inhaled, are similar to those of amyl nitrite.

Who sniffs?

Most first-time sniffers are between 12 and 14, and will have been introduced to sniffing by friends. Sniffing is generally more popular among boys than among girls. Of those:

- 3 out of 4 will try it only once or twice
- 1 in 5 will sniff for a few weeks or months
- 1 in 10 will use solvents long term.

How solvents are used

Generally, some of the inhalant is dropped into a plastic bag or crisp packet and held over the mouth and nose so that the fumes can be inhaled deeply (or 'huffed'). This tends to be a group activity. For more secret sniffing, a liquid that evaporates quickly can be poured on to a rag or a coat sleeve.

Sometimes the user intensifies the experience by inhaling the solvent with his head under the bedclothes or completely inside a plastic bag. In these circumstances, sniffers can suffocate or overdose.

Gas lighter fuel can be sprayed into a balloon or a bag before inhaling. Aerosols and spray paints are usually inhaled directly. A number of people have died through squirting aerosol gases directly into their mouths, freezing their air passages.

The effects

The effects of sniffing are similar to being drunk and include getting a hangover. The inhaled chemicals are rapidly absorbed into the bloodstream, going from the lungs to the brain in a matter of seconds and giving the user a euphoric 'rush'.

These peak effects usually last for only a few minutes or so, and are followed by a relaxed sense of well-being lasting half an hour or more. Some users say that the intensity of the pleasurable effects increases with regular sniffing, but the opposite is more likely to be true.

The bad effects

During the 'high', most users are aware that their heart is pounding faster. About 1 in 3 report unpleasant headaches, buzzing in the ears, and nausea. A few experience chest or stomach pains. Fumes may cause coughing bouts, sneezing, and streaming eyes, and a rash around the mouth and nose.

After the high, users feel depressed and lethargic, irritable and restless, with a poor appetite and altered sleep patterns.

Sniffers can be accidentally injured because they are in an unsafe place—on a roof or by a railway line. Some sniff to the point of unconsciousness and then risk death by choking on their vomit. Strong emotions or physical exercise while using solvents can bring on a heart attack, even in young people, and are thought to be responsible for half solvent-related deaths.

About 150 young people die every year from inhaling solvents, and solvents contribute to more deaths among people under 20 than any other drug. More than 80 per cent of solvent-related deaths occur in this age group, and 60 per cent of these are in young people under 17. Approximately 10 per cent of solvent-related deaths occur in children sniffing for the first time.

Heavy use of solvents is commoner among people who already have psychological problems. There is no evidence that solvent misuse causes mental illness.

Occasional and even regular sniffers do not experience withdrawal symptoms when they stop, apart from a hangover. Very heavy users, however, may experience problems similar to those of people dependent on alcohol—trembling, sweating, and agitation. Heavy solvent misuse can result in lasting damage to the brain. Long-term misuse of aerosols and cleaning fluids has been known to cause lasting kidney, liver and lung damage.

The law

Although it is not illegal to inhale solvents, the Intoxicating Substances Supply Act was introduced in 1985, making it illegal for shopkeepers to sell to under-18s if they know they are under 18 and are going to use the solvents to get high.

Facts:
Alcohol

Alcohol is the drug most commonly used by young people at illegal and legal ages:

- nearly 90 per cent of boys in the UK have drunk alcohol by the age of 13
- alcohol reaches your brain within five minutes of swallowing it
- it is a depressant drug which slows brain activity
- it affects women more quickly than men and the effects last longer
- fizzy drinks increase the speed of absorption of alcohol
- eating before drinking slows the absorption of alcohol
- alcohol affects our sense of right and wrong before it affects our co-ordination
- 25 per cent of 13–17 year-olds get into arguments and fights after drinking alcohol
- 1,000 children under 15 years of age are admitted to hospital each year with acute alcohol poisoning
- 18–24 year-olds are the heaviest drinkers
- people who drink too much in the evening may still be 'over the limit' next morning

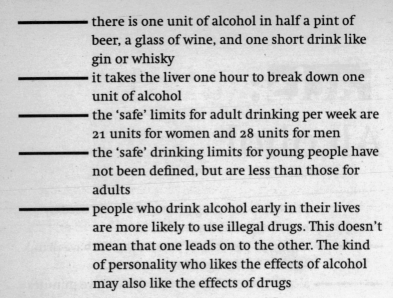

- there is one unit of alcohol in half a pint of beer, a glass of wine, and one short drink like gin or whisky
- it takes the liver one hour to break down one unit of alcohol
- the 'safe' limits for adult drinking per week are 21 units for women and 28 units for men
- the 'safe' drinking limits for young people have not been defined, but are less than those for adults
- people who drink alcohol early in their lives are more likely to use illegal drugs. This doesn't mean that one leads on to the other. The kind of personality who likes the effects of alcohol may also like the effects of drugs

The Drinkline numbers are:

London only: 0171 332 0202

All UK: 0345 32 02 02

All calls are charged at the local rate.

The lines are open:

Monday to Friday 9·30 a.m.–11 p.m.

Saturday and Sunday 6–11 p.m.

There is also a dial and listen 'freecall' service on 0500 801802

Ben regularly takes ecstasy

and occasionally cannabis and amphetamines. He is an unemployed 20-year-old and lost his last job through continually being late in the morning. His parents live in the north of England and he has no contact with them. He shares a flat in a squat in Bristol with his girlfriend, who is waitressing to earn the money to support them both.

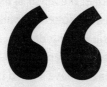

I take ecstasy about once a month. It makes me feel brilliant, euphoric, and like I want to dance. There is a release of stress and hassle—a period of total enjoyment. It takes me about half an hour to come up on the drug. The longest it has ever taken is about an hour and a quarter, but that turned out to be the best E, and lasted the longest.

You get this 'head fuck' when you feel it come on, and it's like you go dizzy. Then it makes you 'rush'. I don't find it a particularly physical thing. It's more like . . . you're looking . . . there's an atmosphere . . . and you see this atmosphere . . . it's just friendliness and emotion.

The physical rushes aren't that severe. Well, I've never found them to be, apart from one time. I think it was in a club in Hull, when I had what is termed a

'Humpty Dumpty'. On that occasion, I found myself all of a sudden just totally off my head. All the blood rushed to the end of my fingers and my hands felt like they were swelling up. Oh, and my hair felt tingly, like someone was gently flicking it all the time. I felt like I was the coolest bastard in the place, that I was totally lost from the rest of the crowd but not isolated.

I think my emotions are the same as everyone else's there, but I don't find it easy to communicate with people who aren't 'off it' when I am. As you come down, that's when the communicating gets easier. You feel very friendly and there is a sensation of allegiance. I think perhaps that is what is meant by 'knowing the score'.

It's hard to say the main reason I take E, but the music is important. The music enhances the drug, and the drug enhances the music. With E, the music is more than just a sound, it's creating the atmosphere. I think I could go into a club and enjoy the music without drugs. I could have a good time and be quite a sexy dancer to boot! Mostly I do drugs because I know I'm going to have a good time with my mates.

I do find I can hallucinate a bit on E, especially this one called a 'snowball', but not half as much as on acid. I don't tend to feel paranoid either, not like the blind panic I've felt on acid. A more common side-effect is that my jaw tenses up and I chew a lot. Yes, I definitely gurn quite a bit. Afterwards, I'm not sleepless as such, but I might keep waking up. This only happens on the night after the E, and it only takes me a day or so to get back to normal sleeping. After I first get up, I feel mellow for the rest of the day.

Although after every drug I've ever taken I've come down feeling 'I liked that and I want to do it again', it's a mental rather than a physical addiction. There's no way I would physically crave an E.

I don't believe reports about people dying after taking just one E. One of my friends died after taking five. He'd only been taking E for a couple of months, and he'd never done more than two, so he'd not built up a resistance. I've known other people take five and be fine. In the newspaper report they said that 'the lad had never taken drugs in his life before,' whereas I know that he was in there selling Es—he was dealing. But he decided to take them instead. The inaccuracies in the report came from his mates trying to protect his mother. They said that he was just having a binge to celebrate the end of his exams, which was crap. When he died, we all said, 'Right, that's it, we're never having Es or speed.' I've started again since, and the lads that used to E with him regularly were 'E'ing the next weekend after he died.

I remember the first time I ever properly took a drug. It was acid, and before I took it I was a bit worried. But when I'd taken it, the thought that stayed with me most was that all that stuff I'd been told in school about it being dangerous was bullshit. If you take drugs in moderation and you're sensible about it, they can be a good experience and not dangerous at all.

With E I do take basic precautions—wear baggy clothes, drink a lot, etcetera. But the media likes to hype these things and make it an emotive subject. Why? Because it sells. People are more keen to read about the relatively low number of deaths on E than about the great time the majority of people are having on it. That Cook report on E, for example, it was just sensationalism—how E steals the lives of defenceless young kids who get forced into taking it! Whoever heard such a thing? No one ever pressured me saying 'do ecstasy', and I never felt obliged to do it just because my friends were. I started doing it because people told me how brilliant it was.

My mate was stupid, and the next day everyone was saying, 'What a stupid twat.' Basically, I'll do most drugs in moderation. But having said that, I have done silly mixers in one night—whizz with poppers with booze with weed, and a dash of coke. So there have been times when I worry I'm going too far. My brother is totally fucked up on drugs and I sometimes find myself slipping to where he is.

I'll grow out of it when the circumstances are right, I'm sure, but I still feel I want to and I need to for a while yet. As far as the risks go, I'm aware of the dangers of potentially overdosing—that it is possible on just one E—but this is relative. I am more concerned about the long-term problems because these are unknown. The sort of thing, you know, like my kids not being quite like human beings! But I know a lot of people who are taking much more than me, and there's a weird security in that.

On New Year's Eve I came in with Mandy and thought, 'It's a bastard, I'm going to have to give this up.' For twenty-four hours I felt like someone had got hold of my heart and was squeezing it as tightly as they could. But I put that down mainly to sniffing poppers at the same time, not down to the actual E.

I don't feel bad about taking it with my mates down here, but there are mates back home who I couldn't even mention the word 'ecstasy' in front of—let alone tell them that I do it. Frankly, they just don't want to know. All in all, in spite of some of the problems associated with E, the gains are worth it compared to never having tried it.

Although I will have weed with E, I don't generally like sedative drugs. I prefer a drug that lifts you up, like whizz or E. But it depends what you are doing. An occasion like going to a club suits doing an E.

I do think drugs in general should be legalized. There would be greater control of E, and it would be cleaner and safer for the user. This would also stop it from coming through criminal channels and improve the money aspect. The big people who are selling E are robbing and thieving. I've never bought an E in a club. I prefer to buy them from people I already know—then I know what I am getting.

The way I perceive drug taking as a whole is this. I've seen a lot of people doing it, and I've seen losers and winners. I've got an uncle and a mate who have died. I've seen others who took way too much, way too often, and have suffered as a consequence. Most of them have permanently got some kind of fuck up in their lives. I've seen mates who looked like they were going to fuck up, but then stopped, and now they are doing OK. But I've also seen people like myself who have taken drugs, and from the start to the present time have done things in moderation, and enjoyed it, and had a good time.

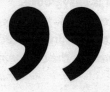

Facts:
Ecstasy

'Dearly beloved,
we are gathered together here today
to get through this thing called life.'
(Prince, 'Let's Go Crazy',
frequently sampled track in the rave scene)

'Your captain tonight is Easygroove.
Please fasten your seat belts,
you are flying with Ecstasy Airways. Let's go!'
(MC announcement at the beginning of a rave,
Universe, 1991)

Ecstasy (MDMA) is a 'hallucinogenic amphetamine' derivative, which means that it affects your mind
and speeds you up. It has become the dance culture drug,
and it is estimated there may be over 500,000 regular users
in Britain.

There have recently been a series of well-publi-
cised deaths of young people which have been associated
with taking ecstasy. In each case various theories have been
put forward as to the cause—the drug was impure; the drug
was too pure; the person had become dehydrated by
drinking too little; the person had become over-hydrated by
drinking too much. However, the exact cause of death asso-

ciated with ecstasy remains, in the majority of cases, unclear—though these dangers definitely need to be acknowledged.

ITS HISTORY

In 1949 the parent drug methylenedioxy-amphetamine (MDA for short) was used in the treatment of Parkinson's disease, without much success. It became known as the 'love drug' and was available on the streets in the UK in the mid-1960s. It was banned in 1971.

The active substance methylenedioxymeth-amphetamine (MDMA for short), which is contained in ecstasy, was synthesised in 1912 and patented in 1914. It was available, quite legally, for recreational use in the USA in the 1970s. In the decade which followed, American psychiatrists were using it successfully as an aid to individual, marital, and group psychotherapy. It was also said to be useful in the treatment of drug and alcohol abuse. It was outlawed in the UK in 1976, but remained legal in the US until 1985.

Towards the end of the 1980s, dedicated night clubbers began hearing wonderful things about ecstasy (E):

'It could even make white men dance—or think they could—unless they went to public school, of course. Nothing can make a toff dance—nothing.'

'Only E could make you move like MC Hammer, talk like you really, really care, sweat like a Sumo wrestler, and pull faces like a champion gurner. A legend was in the making.'

(Lifeline)

THE STUFF ITSELF

There are more than a thousand variations of the basic amphetamine chemical, but by far the most widely used is ecstasy itself (MDMA). Because of its illegal status, little is known in detail about the way it acts on the body. However, the results of an oral dose become apparent within 30 minutes, peak at about 60–90 minutes, and disappear in about 4 hours. MDA (snowballs, white caps) is much less common than ecstasy and is reported to be longer lasting and a rougher ride. It is less euphoric, more amphetamine-like, and towards the psychedelic end of the range. MDEA (Eve) occasionally crops up and is one of the many variants of the basic molecule. MDMA combines the effects of acid and whizz and has been referred to as a 'psychedelic amphetamine'.

Other variants sometimes sold as ecstasy:

LOVE HEARTS = a decongestant

SPLITS = decongestants

WHITE CALLYS = antihistamine

CALIFORNIA SUNRISE = amphetamine/caffeine

GREEN BURGERS = amphetamine/caffeine

Although one analysis of various Es carried out in 1993 found that very few actually contained any MDMA, other seizures revealed high purity. Even so, less than half the drugs bought as E actually are E. The rest are 'snidey'.

Snidey Es range from a bit of E mixed with something else to totally snidey Es which can be dog worming tablets or fish tank cleansers. Most worrying of the ingredients that are being used to 'snidey up' Es are depressants and anaesthetics. Among these, ketamine is the most common. Sedatives (or 'downers') like phenobarbitone have also been found in E.

ITS FORM

Ecstasy comes in tablets and capsules of various shapes, colours and sizes, selling at anything from £12 to £25 each. These have names like DOVES, DENNIS THE MENACE, DISCO BISCUITS, RHUBARB AND CUSTARD,

BURGERS, M25S, and NEW YORKERS. Es are often reffered to simply as 'pills'. The normal MDMA content is between 75 and 200 milligrams. At some nightclubs in Amsterdam it is possible to get the drug tested.

Ecstasy is mainly swallowed but it is also available as a powder and a liquid, and can be snorted or even injected. Its main users have been nightclubbers and ravers, and 'New Agers' seeking enlightenment; but it is also increasingly used by couples and small groups of young people in the same casual way that their parents might have a few drinks. The amphetamine-like effects make it attractive to some people as a slimming aid.

THE EFFECTS

The effects start after about 20 minutes and can last several hours. Heart rate and blood pressure increase. The jaw muscles tighten and users find themselves grinding their teeth ('gurning') and licking their lips. This is followed by 'a rushing sensation like an orgasm that starts at your toes and goes through your body'. There is a feeling of closeness and empathy with other people, but although ecstasy certainly increases the sensual experience of sex, it can cause men to fail to have an erection and delay orgasm in both sexes. Some users have reported more confidence in relating to other people, an increased awareness of their emotions, and less aggressive impulses. Others say that the experience has made them rethink their priorities in life.

Ecstasy is often used in conjunction with 'poppers' for bringing users up, and dope for coming down. Taken in large amounts, the drug can cause feelings of anxiety and confusion, even paranoia.

THE BAD EFFECTS

If Es were made by legal registered chemists,

you would be advised to take no more than 1.5 milligrams per kilo in body weight and no more often than once every six weeks. There is no cast-iron evidence, but it does seem there is a real risk of certain people developing some kind of mental illness from persistent use too often.

The unwanted side-effects include clumsiness and lack of co-ordination, disorientation and poor concentration, and nausea and vomiting if you come up too quickly. Regular use can result in sleep problems and lethargy when the drug wears off. Fits and liver damage have also been reported. And combining E with other illicit or prescribed drugs can prove fatal.

There is a serious risk of dehydration from dancing for hours in a hot and crowded space. In some people the drug itself also causes a rise in body temperature, which can lead to heatstroke, coma, and death. It is very important to drink plenty of water if you are taking Es and partying vigorously. On the other hand, overdoing the water can make your body lose salt, and E itself may heighten this effect: at least one recent death has been attributed to this. Sip water rather than gulp it, and include isotonic sports drinks and salty snacks.

Ecstasy is not physically addictive, but as the drug acts like a stimulant, it is particularly dangerous for those who have a heart condition or suffer from diabetes, asthma or epilepsy. However, although millions of people have taken E on a regular basis, only a relatively small number of deaths have been directly related to its effects.

THE LAW

Ecstasy is a class A drug. It is illegal to possess it. Supplying can land you in jail, and that includes selling it to your friends.

Ian is into the hard stuff.

He is 18 and works in a garage in the East End of London. He still lives at home with his parents, who are aware that he 'puffs' but not that he now has a coke habit.

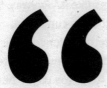

I started to puff out of boredom and curiosity. All my mates smoked, and there were three or four dealers on my block, so I thought, 'Why not?' There seemed to be more reason to do it than not to do it.

I remember looking at things and cracking up laughing, and I couldn't feel the floor. I think that's why people call it 'getting high'! Then I remember seeing a police car and getting para—walking a bit faster and then running. I think my mum and dad found out when I came home and my mum made me some Ovaltine. I was so stoned I forgot I hated it and drank the lot. They knew I was on something then.

What we'd do when we got home after a puff is the 'red eye test' and the 'deep and meaningful test' to make sure we could carry through a conversation with the old man. For a long time my mum and dad didn't know I did it regular. They'd rather turn a blind eye than think I was actually taking drugs. When I started to grow my own hemp plants in my mum's window boxes, she thought they were weeds and tore them up. I went crazy, but I couldn't say anything—it was terrible.

I used to skin up in front of my mum and she'd assume it was a fag. When I was 17 I did manage to get my mum to puff, and she will do it on occasions. Last Christmas she put it in the gravy, and Gran was off her face. Everyone was in hysterics, we couldn't breathe we were laughing so much. It was a good Christmas! In fact, it turned into a bit of a bad Oxo habit. I just couldn't keep my hands off it! There's a saying, 'If you give up drink, drugs and sex, you don't live longer—it just seems like it.' Anyway, Mum's the addict. She can't wake up without a cup of tea.

The best thing about getting stoned is the 'munchies'. Strawberry milkshake is my favourite. When you're tripping, you don't eat food 'cos you're hungry. You do it 'cos of the smell and the texture. I had this kebab, and it was like the best food I'd ever had, but the next bite I was nearly sick on it. I was so disappointed. I used to go home and raid the cupboards—not to eat stuff but just to feel it.

I generally 'mong out' on puff. It gives me a different perspective on things. Take that poster over there. It don't mean much on its own, but if you were buzzing you'd be a part of it. It's like when people are talking to you normal it don't mean much, but when you're stoned, it's like world importance. And then you get these pointless arguments like who's going to make the tea. Or who's going to get some Rizla and ten Bennies (Benson and Hedges). They go on for hours till someone does the honourable thing. Once we had to chip in and pay a mate a tenner to go across the road and buy a packet of Rizla. Puffing does make you slack.

A lot of times we have to puff outside, but a proper

session will be in a small room—bit of music, bucket bong, couple of beers. That will last hours till about six in the morning. If we didn't have a bong, we used to get my brother's motor-cycle helmet, put it on, and get blowbacks into it through a crack in the visor. People would always come out green from that. Once my mate threw up in it. It was horrid, man. I spent the rest of the night cleaning it out, because there was no way I was explaining that one to my brother.

When we only had a couple of spliff's worth, we used to do it in the phone box—'cos everyone got to breathe in the smoke. We'd get about five of us in there. I remember opening the doors and all the smoke pouring out—it looked like the bleeding Tardis. Also, we used to do it against the speakers. We'd put a really bassy tune on, so the cone was moving, give it a blowback, and breathe in the smoke as the cone went in and out.

But puff has shot my memory. When I'm caned, I'll start making a cup of tea and then forget what I'm doing. Once after this spliff, I decided I needed to get something, so I walked three miles into town, but when I got there I couldn't remember what I'd come for, and I had to turn around and walk all the way back.

The next thing we did was tripping—that was wicked. Fags never tasted like fags, they were whatever flavour you wanted—I had weed, hash, toffee apple and chocolate. When I started on magic mushrooms and acid, I was hallucinating. It should have been scary, but I was just laughing about it. As long as you know it's just the drug doing it, it's all right. Doing mushrooms was great. I thought I was Sonic the Hedgehog, and I was going round collecting rings all night. But my stomach was always done in the next day, and my shit was like mango sauce.

I was 16 when I first tried acid—which I wouldn't do

now. I think it's better taken with an innocent mind when you're young and your thoughts are unstructured. Otherwise it's dangerous. I have a friend who's taken acid and he now has a permanently altered perception of life. He ended up in the mental hospital, and although he's all right now he will never be the same again. They say that no one is ever quite the same after their first trip.

I had a trip once and as I was coming down, I got quite para because of what someone said. They just said, 'Shut up,' casual like, and I took it really personal. I have another mate who lost it bad on acid, though it was the bucket bong that pushed him over the edge. He thought he'd died, and we spent ages convincing him not to call his Muslim parents at four o'clock in the morning to tell them what Mecca was like!

The first time I had acid I went to a Grateful Dead concert. I stupidly took two and promptly lost the plot. But then, Grateful Dead concerts are mad environments anyway. On the way home, I didn't know when I was going to come down off it, and I says to my mate, 'Look, there's a dead Doberman in the road.' It was only when we went right up to it I realized it was a dustbin liner. Then I knew I was tripping. Now I often look at people and think, 'Thank the fuck I'm not tripping now.'

The next drug I tried was coke, but that was by accident. This bloke offered me a spliff in a nightclub, and when I tasted it, it was really sweet. When I asked him what it was, he said, 'Co-coaaina.' I said, 'What?', and he said, 'Cocaine.' It's a sad fact, but now I'm on coke and I can't get off.

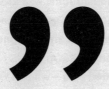

Facts:
Psychedelics and hallucinogens

'If I was fully dosed on psychedelics and tried to play . . . guitar strings would turn to rubber, my hands would pass entirely through the instrument, and the audience (if I saw them at all) could be anything from a field of waving buttercups to a pack of howling demons.'
(David Crosby, guitarist/songwriter with Crosby, Stills, Nash & Young in the late 60s)

LSD, Magic Mushrooms, PCP

'In a dreamlike state, with eyes closed, I perceived an uninterrupted stream of fantastic pictures, extraordinary shapes with intense kaleidoscopic play of colours.'
(Albert Hoffman, discoverer of LSD)

Their history

Highly toxic mescal beans, psilocybin mushrooms, and the mescaline contained in the tips of the Peyote cactus were used ritually in the Americas thousands of years before the birth of Christ.

However, it wasn't until 1943, when Albert Hoffman, a research scientist, accidentally ingested a small amount of a chemical he had been researching as a new heart stimulant that psychedelic drugs hit the Western world.

Feeling odd after taking this first accidental dose, Hoffman explored further. He took what he thought was a tiny dose (250 micrograms) of the substance he labelled lysergic acid diethylamide-25 (LSD). As anything over 50 micrograms has a hallucinatory effect, the ensuing 'trip' was powerful!

Subsequently, the Central Intelligence Agency (CIA) in the States took a strong interest in the drug, using it for interrogation and the reprogramming of those who had been brainwashed. Many army personnel, prisoners, autistic children and psychiatric patients were given LSD without their knowledge or their consent—resulting in at least one death. A man threw himself out of a window while in the grip of a prolonged psychotic state a week after receiving the drug.

Writers such as Aldous Huxley, Ken Kesey, Allen Ginsberg, and William Burroughs became regular users of hallucinogens, along with jazz musicians such as Thelonius Monk, Dizzy Gillespie, and John Coltrane. In 1960, a Harvard professor, Timothy Leary, took psilocybin mushrooms and 'was swept over the edge of a sensory Niagara into a maelstrom of transcendental visions and hallucinations'. His catchphrase, 'turn on, tune in, drop out', became the mantra for the sixties generation.

Lysergic acid diethylamide (LSD)

LSD (also known as acid) is a white, tasteless powder which dissolves easily in water. It is usually sold as a liquid, impregnated into small squares of blotting paper or card and then dissolved on the tongue. These squares often carry colourful abstract designs or pictures of cartoon or film characters such as the Pink Panther. The designs are used as trade names, such as STRAWBERRIES or CHINESE DRAGON.

LSD is relatively cheap at about £4 a trip, and it is highly potent. The problem is that you never know how much actual LSD you are getting.

The effects

The effects can begin within 20 minutes, peak at around 2–3 hours, and last for 8 hours or longer. Users have an 'out of body' mystical experience in which colours intensify, moving objects leave tracks, patterns appear and disappear. Vision, hearing and touch are all distorted, but users usually remain aware that this is the effect of the drug.

Nobody has died from an LSD overdose, but fatal accidents under the influence do occur. Prolonged depression or psychosis is unusual if there has been no previous history of mental illness or personality problems. Psychological dependence is very rare. Sensitivity to the drug rapidly decreases but returns if you don't take it for a while.

The bad effects

A bad trip can cause anxiety, paranoia, fear, and nasty hallucinations. It is inadvisable to take LSD if you are feeling depressed, and the effects take a long time to wear off. The drug interferes with judgement and concentration, which has resulted in fatal accidents. It has also, very rarely, led to suicide.

If you do try LSD, leave sufficient time free (12 to 24 hours to cope with the effects), and have a friend around to reassure you in case you start to panic. You should not take LSD if you have a psychiatric illness.

The law

LSD is a class A drug. You can get up to 7 years for possession and life imprisonment for supplying.

Magic Mushrooms

'Magic mushrooms' grow wild in damp fields and heaths in the UK between September and November. Their use goes back thousands of years to when ancient peoples took them in quests for spiritual enlightenment. They were adopted in the West in the 1960s, as a natural alternative to LSD.

The popular name for the most common kind is 'Liberty Cap', a white and rocket shaped mushroom. It is very hard to tell one mushroom from another and if you pick the wrong one, you can poison yourself. Even the right one can give you stomach ache as well as hallucinations.

The strength of the hallucinations depends on how many mushrooms you eat. They can be eaten raw, cooked, or stewed into a tea or infusion. The effects of a mushroom trip are similar to an acid one, but usually less intense and shorter lasting.

There is no law against eating magic mushrooms raw, and enough for a mild trip (about 30) can be bought for a few pounds. It is illegal, however, to 'make them into a preparation'.

Phencyclidine (PCP)

PCP (known as 'angel dust') was marketed in the 1950s as an anaesthetic, but was soon restricted and was withdrawn completely in 1965 because of its severe side-effects. It is a very strong painkiller that both depresses and stimulates the brain at the same time.

PCP is usually smoked, though some people stir it into a drink, others snort it, and the lunatic fringe inject it. It produces hallucinatory effects that last about 4 hours and are followed by a longer period of irritable depression.

PCP has never really taken off in the UK, although it and ketamine are widely reported as ingredients of 'snidey' ecstasy and 'snidey' hash. In a recent survey, 14 out of 100 people whose urine tested positive for PCP were unaware that they had taken it.

Ketamine (K)

Ketamine ('Special K', 'Super K' or 'K') is a derivative of PCP and was developed in the early 1960s as an anaesthetic. Its use is on the up among those who have tired of E and are looking for new drug experiences. It is sold as red and white or gold and white capsules, or white tablets and powder, for between £6 and £25 a 'hit'. It is either swallowed or injected.

K is quicker acting and safer than its parent, but the effects are more intense. It removes you from reality and yourself and also acts as a painkiller. Disorientation and confusion commonly occurs.

Not everybody enjoys the ketamine experience. People talk about nightmare hallucinations, tunnel vision, blackouts, memory loss, and thinking they were going to die. Ketamine also stimulates the cardiovascular system, which can cause high blood pressure and a potentially dangerous increase in heart rate.

Strictly speaking, ketamine is not illegal, though as it is normally used only for medical and veterinary purposes, you might have to answer a few questions about where you obtained your supply!

Gammahydroxybutyrate (GHB, more often known as GBH)

GBH, which was also originally developed as an anaesthetic, is a relatively recent arrival. It is a colourless, odourless liquid which is taken by mouth and is also available in powder and capsule form. Its street price ranges from £5 for a capful to £10–15 for a bottle.

The effects of GBH are described as a cross between LSD and ecstasy. The drug takes effect in anything from 10 minutes to an hour, and has been reported to last as long as a day. In small doses, it breaks down inhibitions and increases your sex drive. Its bad effects include nausea, vomiting, stiffening of muscles, convulsions, coma, and failure to breathe. So far, however, there have been no confirmed deaths.

The law
GBH is not illegal at the moment.

John will try anything.

He is 18 and went to a minor public school. He was asked to leave when it was discovered he had been smoking cannabis with three of his friends. He is now working in a wine store, but is hoping to go into the City as a shares dealer.

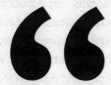

I started smoking cigarettes long before puff. I used to bunk off school and do it for the buzz. I first had puff when I was 14 or 15. By then, everyone was puffing and I was buying half ounces. My experience of drugs at school was not good. My friends had started puffing before me, but I'd started smoking cigarettes before them, so I was quite cool on that front.

One day a friend had some spliffs he was selling for £2 each, which was a rip-off, but I remember buying them in order to celebrate the end of GCSEs. We went into this disused room and hid in there and smoked them. Then we went into the common room to have some tea, and I was so fucked I lost it. I went really white, I was shaking, I was weak. I didn't know where I was, I was talking shit. I had people coming up to me saying, 'What's wrong with you?', and my mates were just laughing. This made it worse because serious paranoia then kicks in.

They got a bit worried about me after a while and took me to the medical room, and then I was really paranoid! They called the headmaster, and the next thing I hear is his booming voice shouting from the corridor: 'Reed!' I should have known he was calling to another student about the 'no running' sign, but I thought he'd said 'weed' and was referring to me! I was terrified.

I got thrown out for that. I didn't think it was fair, but the school had 'a policy'. I think it was to satisfy all the rich parents that they were 'doing something about the drug problem.' What they were 'doing' was me! We'd been boozing a lot at school as well, plus Tipp-Ex thinner and a bit of glue at the back of the maths class. That was a big thing too. I got nicked the next year going to Glastonbury with a half, and went to court the next morning. We got fined £100.

We used to bong up on oil after that—a class 'A', I think. If it's not, it should be. I had a trip about then too, a black microdot—it was great. We all went up to the heath, just clocking the sunrise over the hill, throwing yellow daffodils up against the purple sky—you know the scene.

I've had an 'out of body' experience on mushrooms. We did a brew of fresh ones, and drank the lot, not really knowing how much to take. On top of that, I had some of my friend's bong. We called it 'the beast 10', as it was about a metre long. We boshed two grams each of the beast 10, and then we went downstairs. My friend put this video on, where there's just these white lines that spiral across the screen. The whole room went white and we took off. There were spheres and tubes and pyramids and triangles, all different shapes and colours, and all me and my friend said to each other was the occasional tentative, 'Are you like just tripping off your nut?' Just as it was starting to get light, we suddenly went 'click' and came out of it simultaneously. He looks at me and says, 'Shall we go?' I say, 'Yeah,' and we were out of there. He went one way, I went the other.

Another time there was a bunch of us doing a cocktail of drugs, and the guy next to me passed me a 'J'. As I was puffing on it, I saw something coming out of his mouth, but I carried on anyway. Then he started shaking a bit, and I thought he was messing around and told him to stop. He started shaking more before having a full-scale epileptic fit. He was all right in the end, but I've never sobered up so quickly in my life.

I like Es, though I find that and speed shrivel your dick up a bit. It's like you go for a pee and you've lost it. You're thinking, 'I'm sure I used to have one.' We would bosh a few Es, and take some amyl, and then go to raves. On the way back, we'd have people skinning up in the car, but I used to worry about the butts and the hot rocks, because I've got burn holes all over my clothes. I'd get them to lob the butts out of the window. Well, this one must have blown back in and into the boot. There we were, all chilled out after a good night, and I looked in the mirror and there's flames coming out of where the spare tyre should have been. Everyone did the most rational thing and panicked. We managed to get it out though, with the water from the hubbly-bubbly.

Driving on drugs is always a funny one. I think that I'm far safer than normal, because I always overcompensate. Once we went to this rave and I was driving on an E, acid, spliffs, Valium, and some whizz. At the end of the journey, one of my friends remarked that he'd been convinced he'd been travelling in the Star Ship *Enterprise* and I was Captain Kirk. I felt complimented, but a little unsure whether or not to confess that I had felt the same way.

Driving on drugs, I often think I'm in a simulation machine playing 'pole position', and having to remind myself that, unlike in the game, you only get one life.

On Valium, my best friend got this idea of throwing his bike in the Thames to collect on the insurance, so we lobbed it off the bridge. Two days later, he came back from school and it had returned from the dead. It was sitting in the garden with weeds all over it and a note from his mum saying, 'Next time you decide to throw your bike in the river, let the tyres down.'

The thing I really got into was speed. I call some drugs 'ladders' because you come up gently in small steps, like with puff or booze. Then there's 'creepers' that creep up on you and then hit you—boom and you peak fast. Speed's like that. First time I had a gram, I remember drinking loads of Lucosade Sport. That's a bit like speed. I was thinking, 'Have I come up yet?', and then boom—cold sweat pouring down my face and rushing like a nutter. I was hot and then cold and I felt all tingly. Music's amazing on speed. I used to love Jungle, but then I got much more into House and Happy Hardcore. It's something me and my friends always argue about.

When we started to cocktail our drugs, we'd have uppers and then downers, and mix them depending on what mood we were in. We'd create new names for the different drugs. Trips we'd call 'wows', because everything's 'wow' when you're tripping. We'd call cannabis 'sketchy', because everything's sketchy like a notebook—a bit hazy, or we'd call it 'bungle', because when we have it everything is 'bungly'. All my mates use nicknames like that.

We'd talk about all sorts when we were stoned, usually big things we didn't understand, like the stars and the supernatural. When we first took drugs, we used to talk about the different feelings we'd get. One of them is a 'circle' feeling in the stomach, when you want to laugh, you want to eat, and you want something else but you don't know what it is.

I hate bright lights when I'm on drugs, so I usually carry dark glasses with me and I wear them in McDonald's when I'm stoned. When I'm tripping, I have a special tripping hat. I call it my safety hat, because it stops my brain escaping.

There's a few good films I've seen recently that I like to watch on drugs, like *The Doors* and *Wayne's World* and *Pulp Fiction*. The most headspin one I ever saw was *Jacob's Ladder*. It's a true story about these American troops in Korea who were given twenty times the normal dose of acid, without them knowing, to make them into killing machines—the principle being that you return to your most basic human instinct—to defend.

I like using drugs to suit my mood—they can take me in whatever direction I want. On an average night, I binge Es or ice with amyl nitrite, followed by tranx and spliffs. At three in the morning, it's easier to get drugs than booze.

One time, I was just getting into a trip with my girlfriend—looking at pictures, catching each other's glances, giggling—and I went to bed with her. But I couldn't sort it out, we just kept laughing at my penis, it seemed ridiculous at the time. Mind you, after that, when we started taking Es, sex coming down off them was flipping amazing. In fact once I passed out! I didn't take any more until I started getting into the House scene, when there was this boom in ecstasy, speed, trips, the lot. Those were the best days. We would drive out to free parties, everyone meeting up, no one knowing the location. I got a bit too into those. I was up and down like a yo-yo.

I even took my A levels from my crammers on whizz. I stayed up all the night before, boshed two wraps, had a line before going in, and sniffed the whole way through. I thought I'd done well in those exams. I thought I was up for the Nobel Prize. I was writing at 100 miles per hour. But I only got one D in the end.

One night after an E, speed, booze, and a trip, we all decided to bosh some downers. We had loads of tranx because a friend used to get them on a false prescription— DF118s, mogadons—and we'd have spliff as well. As a group in one room, we'd mong and gauge out. We'd be half-awake and half-asleep and have ridiculous conversations.

I got heavily into Valium last year. I think that was more addictive than toot and I found it very harrowing to come off. I took so many on Christmas Eve that I was found mashed out on Christmas Day, face down in the Christmas tree. But I got caught out when this telephone conversation I had with a friend, about palthium and diamorphine, was recorded on my dad's voice-activated dictaphone.

Ever since then, my dad's been a bit suspicious when I've been home. The other morning when I was half-awake, I caught him out of the corner of my eye testing some sugar left on my floor the night before. I had a chat with him after that, and he confessed that he'd once had mescaline and some coke. First he thought he was Mick Jagger's mother, and then Mum found him in the fridge thinking he was a turkey. He said if he wasn't one then, he certainly felt like one afterwards.

I tried heroin after that, with a group of people they called the 'Silver Beards'. When they took it, their heads would be hanging like an unnecessary accessory to their necks—eyes rolled back, gauched out, mumbling some-thing occasionally, foil in one hand, tube in the other. The first time I took it, I just went green and threw up. After that, it was nice, too nice. It's a most mellow, chill feeling—a little vacation.

One of the main reasons I started on heroin was its accessibility. The addiction creeps up on you. It comes from the core. You melt on the inside first, and then on the outside, not the other way around. Initially, I thought I wasn't getting addicted, until it got like it is with fags—every time I had a problem, I would reach for it. I always thought I was mentally strong before I developed the habit, but in the end I couldn't say 'no'. It seduces you like a *femme fatale*.

Another reason I started was because in the circle of friends I associated with it was the norm. But I could never bring myself to inject. To me, that always seemed the final line you shouldn't cross. The only reason I could maintain the habit was because I was working. Otherwise I would have had to deal to support it. I was spending at least £200 a week.

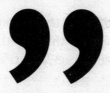

Facts:
Amphetamines

'I would like to suggest that you don't use speed, and here is why: it will mess up your liver, your kidneys, rot out your mind; in general, the drug will make you just like your parents.'

(Frank Zappa)

In the UK, the use of speed (amphetamine) is second only to the use of cannabis. By the time they are 19, at least 10 per cent of the population have tried it at least once.

Its history

Amphetamines were discovered in 1887 by a German physicist, but they were not tested on humans until the 1920s. They were first marketed as a nasal decongestant, then as a treatment for asthma, obesity, narcolepsy (falling asleep all the time) and depression.

Their first non-medical application was to combat tiredness among soldiers in the Second World War. After the war they remained easily available on prescription, but there was a crackdown in 1964 after press reports about the use of amphetamine pills by Mods to fuel all night raving.

Regular users became known as 'speed freaks' or 'whizz heads'. A growing black market developed in amphetamine sulphate (BENNIES), dexamphetamine (DEXIES), methylphenidate (RIT), methylamphetamine (METHS, CRYSTAL), and Durophet (BLACK BOMBERS). A particular favourite among the Mods was Drinamyl (PURPLE HEARTS), a potentially lethal combination of amphetamines and barbiturates.

Its names

Although there is this wide variety of amphetamines, the one you are most likely to come across is amphetamine sulphate, also known as SPEED, UPPERS, SULPHATE, SULPH, WHIZZ, LEAPERS, and BILLY.

Its various forms

Amphetamine sulphate comes in the form of a white powder, frequently mixed with other substances such as bicarbonate of soda and caster sugar. What you buy on the street may be only about 6 per cent amphetamine. It is sold in small paper packets for £10–15 per gram, and is usually snorted, stirred into a drink, rubbed into your gums, or dissolved in water and injected.

The effects

Speed makes you feel self-confident, alert, powerful and energetic. It keeps you going for a long time without food or sleep, but then you collapse and have to catch up with both.

The bad effects

The chemical effects of speed are very similar to those of cocaine, though with speed they last much longer. Experienced users often can't tell the drugs apart.

Speed raises your blood pressure and severely reduces your calcium levels. Because street amphetamines are cut with everything under the sun, those who inject them frequently soon end up in a real mess. Sniffing damages your nose, and rubbing it into your gums can cause your teeth to fall out because of loss of dentine. Pregnant women should avoid it completely. Interactions with certain prescribed medicines can be very dangerous.

Heavy users suffer from disturbed sleep, loss of appetite, uncomfortable itching, and feelings of acute anxiety or paranoia. Irritability and aggression are common. Fits have been reported.

Large doses of amphetamine can cause a complete mental breakdown. It is very addictive, and regular users need bigger and bigger doses to get an effect. Addicts who give up are prone to severe depression.

The law

Speed is normally a class B drug, but if it is prepared for injection it becomes class A, with penalties of up to 5 years in prison for possession, and up to 14 years in prison and an unlimited fine for supplying.

Facts:
Tranquillizers and sleeping pills

Barbiturates

Their history

By the late 1960s, there were more than 2,000 barbiturate-related deaths each year in Britain. Victims worldwide included Brian Jones, Jimi Hendrix, Janis Joplin, and possibly Elvis Presley. At least a third of those attending a London clinic for heroin addicts were regularly injecting barbiturates. And these drugs were second only to the gas oven as a means of committing suicide.

Their names

Barbiturates are also known as BARBS, BLUES, REDS, and SEKKIES.

Their form

Barbiturates, or 'downers', are used to calm people down and are taken as sleeping pills. Most come in powdered form and are sold in coloured capsules. Misusers swallow them, sometimes with alcohol, and inject them.

They are not easily available to street drug users because only limited quantities are manufactured now, but they are still prized by a small minority of oblivion seekers. Dealers often cut barbs into inferior heroin, to give it more potency. Injecting barbs is particularly dangerous.

The effects

A small dose of barbiturates produces a sense of calm and relaxation comparable to a couple of pints of beer. But even modest doses can cause clumsiness, slurred speech, quivering pupils and emotional instability. With regular use the dose tends to grow and there is a danger of physical as well as mental dependence.

The only current medical use for barbs is for treating epilepsy or severe insomnia.

The bad effects

The emotional state of long-term users of barbiturates is characterized by switches from euphoria to depression or irritability, with little warning or provocation.

If barbs are injected, tissue damage can be severe, and because of the rapid destruction of superficial veins, users may be forced to use the large veins in the groin or the neck, with disastrous consequences.

Sudden withdrawal produces anxiety, agitation, trembling, stomach cramps, and sleeplessness. The sufferer may vomit and develop a fever. There is a serious risk of fits which will be difficult to bring under control. Withdrawal should be carried out under medical supervision.

Overdose is very likely to cause interference with the breathing mechanism which can prove fatal.

Benzodiazepines

Benzodiazepines ('bens', or 'benzos') are also prescribed by doctors to control anxiety and tension or to help people to sleep, and have now largely supplanted barbiturates. There is growing concern, however, at both the legal and illegal use of bens, and a growing dependence and misuse has led to a gradual decline in prescriptions.

The different types

There is a wide range of different bens on the market: ... short acting (TEMAZEPAM, OXAZEPAM, LOPRAZOLAM)

... medium acting (LORAZEPAM, ALPRAZOLAM)

... long acting (NITRAZEPAM, DIAZEPAM, KETAZOLAM).

Well-known bens include VALIUM, ATIVAN and LIBRIUM. These drugs are meant to be prescribed for only a few weeks to help cope with a crisis. However, over 250,000 people in the UK have regular prescriptions for them, some stretching over several years. It is easy to become psychologically dependent on bens, and people who try to stop may suffer very unpleasant withdrawal symptoms.

Their availability

Bens are commonly found in medicine cabinets, making it easy for young people to experiment with them. The price on the black market is variable, but cheap. Even on a bad day, £1 will buy 3–4 Diazepam or Temazepam tablets.

The effects

With modest doses, the pleasurable effects of bens are similar to those of alcohol. They take away the worries of life, but they also tend to slow you down, so they reduce alertness and affect the skills where concentration is required, such as driving.

The bad effects

Dependence is fairly common among long-term users, and when people stop taking the drug, they can feel confused, irritable and anxious, and unable to carry out their normal routine.

There is also a risk of overdose, especially if bens are taken with alcohol.

The current most fashionable street ben is Temazepam.

Temazepam

Its names

Temazepam is legal when given on prescription, and is used to help people to sleep. Its street name is JELLIES because in one of its forms it looks like gelatine jelly babies. It is also called WOBBLIES or EGGS.

Its forms

The drug, which is normally swallowed, has until recently been available in two forms: a soft green gelatine capsule containing 20 milligrams of the drug or a white tablet containing 10 milligrams. Some drug takers melt the gelatine capsule into liquid form and inject it directly into their veins, and for this reason capsules have now been withdrawn from sale.

Temazepam is available through dealers, by forging prescriptions, or by buying prescriptions from people who have obtained them legally from a doctor. It is used as a recreational drug by clubbers as a comedown after taking uppers like amphetamines. Others may use it more regularly as an alternative to cannabis, or may inject it in combination with heroin or other drugs. It is not unusual for users to take six or seven capsules at a time—three times the maximum recommended dose.

The effects

Legally used as a sleeping pill, the drug acts as a sedative, taking away worries and fears and bringing on a sense of pleasant relaxation known as being 'monged'. The effects last several hours. Taken with alcohol, Temazepam accentuates the effects of the drink. Prolonged use leads to dependence, especially for those who already have a history of drug abuse.

The bad effects

Injecting the drug is extremely dangerous. This is likely to cause blood clotting, in addition to all the other dangers of injecting drugs, which include blood infections, HIV, and hepatitis. Injected alone, or in various combinations with other drugs, Temazepam has been associated with many deaths.

Sudden withdrawal can cause sweating, depression, nervousness, irritability, and diarrhoea.

The law

The production of the gelatine capsule has now been banned, but the tablets will probably continue to be available on prescription.

Temazepam is now a class B drug. People possessing it without a valid doctor's prescription will be liable for up to 2 years in jail and/or an unlimited fine. Dealing now carries a maximum 5 years in jail and/or an unlimited fine.

Other tranquillizers

There are a number of drugs that are not barbs or bens but have similar effects.

Ethchlorvynol (Placidyl)

A tranquillizer with a characteristic mint-like after-taste. The effects come on about 30 minutes after swallowing the drug, peak after 90 minutes, and last for 4–6 hours. A hangover the next day is quite normal, and the drug has undesirable effects similar to those of barbs.

Glutethimide (Doriden)

This drug enters the brain rapidly, but is broken down in the body rather slowly. In addition to normal barb effects, it can—according to a 1940s article—make you 'hot as a hare, blind as a bat, dry as a bone and mad as a hen.'

Methaqualone (Quaalude, 'Mandrax')

This was withdrawn from legal supply some time ago, but is still highly prized on the black market. The drug is famed for its ability to produce a dreamy 'dissociative high' without sedation—an effect similar to that of heroin. It has, however, been associated with a number of deaths.

Prozac

Prozac is the brand name of fluoxetine hydrochloride, which is a new anti-depressant drug. It is different from many other anti-depressants because it lacks a sedative effect. Users claim that not only does it lift their depression, but it makes them feel 'better than well'.

Prozac is of interest to illegal drug users because it acts on the same part of the brain as E. But mixing Es and Prozac can be dangerous, and has not been shown to either enhance the effects of Es or deal with the side-effects.

Like all drugs, Prozac can cause a range of unwanted effects, and allergic reactions can occasionally be life-threatening. One reported effect common to other anti-depressants is that it can completely ruin your sex life.

According to the experts, 'having a normal person take Prozac is like tuning up a car that is already in tune . . . if something isn't broken, don't try and mend it.'

The law

It is not illegal to possess tranquillizers, but it is illegal to give them away or sell them—and that includes giving away a few tablets from a prescription.

Sara is a crack addict.

She is unemployed and living in a squat. She does not want any details given about her, other than those provided below.

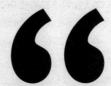

I started puffing when I was 14, and I've been trying to attain that first buzz ever since. But then, the first time I puffed I had seventeen blowbacks. Then I got into the rave scene, and I would be doing up to five or six Es a night. But there were people around me who would be giving it, 'I just dropped my tenth E.' Afterwards we would all go back to a mate's house and come down with lots of blow and videos.

I know people who lick the rock and, like Es, I've seen what it can do. One minute they're genuine good friends and then you never see them again, except to borrow money. I tried it and I must admit, it is a good buzz. It lasts about five minutes, but the thing is, you go so high for such a brief amount of time and then it bangs you right down afterwards. You need it again just to get you close to normality. People will go straight out and nick to order—cars, stereos, phones, whatever. Sometimes, they just put a brick through a window—'smash and grab'.

Most of the crime around here is crack related. That's what all the helicopters up there are about. In fact nowadays, if my mates get stopped with weed, the pigs just throw it away. They're not bothered about it, because there's so much more hard stuff about. The drugs they're really bothered about are the ones that threaten them, like PCP. I saw a bird beat up two coppers on that.

I do whizz as well, but I get more and more pissed off with that because it's full of Ajax. But when it's pure, it's one of the most powerful drugs in the world. I can keep going for days on one fat line of pure whizz. That's one to be careful about though. People don't think of it as being addictive, but I've seen girls as thin as rakes prostitute themselves for it. I saw one bloke, he was about 18, who had no teeth left because he'd been rubbing it so much on his gums.

Trips just make me laugh and laugh. Once I couldn't stop for three days. I know one bloke who got spiked with seven trips. He was a top student but he was never the same again. His life went to ruins. I got spiked once too, but I ended up thanking the geezer because I had a wicked time. When I was on the streets, the boys I met were always trying to get me on trips to confuse me into bed, but I would have none of it—it was money or nothing.

There's a lot of needles on the street and a lot of people offering you 'brown'. I threw up the first time. But when I was on the streets, it was drink I got most into. Booze was good because it sort of numbs you. To get out of that, I had to move town and leave all my friends, because like with any drug, when you give it up you have to give up the whole social aspect that goes with it. I was 13 when I started drinking, and by the age of 16 I was a registered alcoholic. Part of the reason I started was because of what my step-dad used to do to me, and he was an alcho. I also wanted to prove that you could go out on the booze and not get aggro.

At my worst, I was on three bottles of Smirnoff a day and the beers. I came off with spliff, mainly because that helped with the comedowns when I was fully 'clucking'. First there is the physical thing, and at times your whole body will be shaking; and then there is the depression. I tried to commit suicide twice coming off the booze.

I used to do a bit of joyriding when we were on drugs, but it was mainly ram-raiding or car popping to fund the next buzz. See, if you're not buzzing, there's nothing else to do. I got caught one day nicking this nice motor — alloys, boss stereo, the lot. We used to have this special tool to put on the locks. It'd open them in seconds. But there was this one time when I got in, the locks clicked shut all round and I was trapped.

Some boys came out of a van next to me, got into the car and said I was now to work with them. They'd supply the equipment and fake licences and they'd give me a set rate on each car. It was one of their cars and they'd set me up.

They also gave me large amounts of hash to knock out on tick. By doing that, they knew they had people by the balls. At the time I thought it was great. They were looking after me and if I had any trouble they would sort it out. I was living large for a while. I must have been one of the richest girls in the area. I could buy as much booze and drugs as I wanted. After a while, though, I wanted out. I could see it was all leading to big trouble and I didn't want to be beholden to them for the rest of my life.

The only way I could get out was to go homeless. I've seen what they do to people who try to leave or who don't pay their debts. There was this one time when a boy who'd been given a nine-bar on tick hadn't paid up in a month. They put him in the back of this car I'd just nicked, and the next thing was they'd slashed his face and chucked him out of the car at 50 miles per hour.

Going back to crack. The first time I scored some was in the middle of winter outside this club. I was shivering like fuck, and after he'd delivered some stuff, this guy said to me, 'You look cold.' I told him I was and he gave me his leather jacket. I thought it was a pick-up and said, 'Thanks. How d'you know you'll see me again?' He just said, 'You'll be back.'

I was. I tried a little bit of what was in one of the pockets and I tell you, I went up so high it was unbelievable. The feeling I got was like all the drugs I'd ever had all in one go. I was up for about three minutes, then I levelled out for a couple more and came down. The buzz was short but so sweet.

I didn't lick the rock again for about a month. After that I was doing it about four times a week. I had a mild habit but I was spending about £300 a week, and that's low for a crackhead. The temptation to do it again is enormous—especially when you know you can get it twenty-four hours a day. I've got twenty quid in my pocket now. I could call a few numbers and get some rocks delivered by BMW in a matter of minutes.

The main reason you do it again is the comedown. If you are lucky you can sleep it off, but there is still a lot going on in your heart and in your head. I can't really explain the emotion coming down, because you don't feel anger or sorrow. You think about the money you have spent, and the fact that you will be trying to do the same again in a couple of days.

The worst thing is the money you spend on it. I'd come home with £50 in my pocket. £40 would go on rocks, and the other £10 on food, living off bread and baked beans for the rest of the week. It makes you desperate. One day in my squat I found a rock on the table. It wasn't mine, but I slipped it into my sock and tried to make off with it. I got caught and nearly got my head kicked in. I've met a lot of people on rocks who would smoke, and then for the next rock would go out and nick something to sell.

We had people offering us guns and £400 stereos and Technics turntables for £40 quid. It was tempting to buy this stuff, but I would rather have spent the money on rocks as well, and they'd probably have nicked it all back off us in a couple of days.

I've seen crackheads as young as 14. You can spot them because of the look in their eyes—sort of glazed and focused beyond you. But it's a look you can only really recognize having had it yourself.

I was in the shopping centre the other day and there was three 12 to 14-year-old kids trying to hold me up with a Stanley knife. Now I'm big and heavy, with a skinhead at the moment, so if I get threatened there has to be a crack problem. I see it happen in the clubs, but it's hard to find the dealers because they've got runners working for them. The dealers are clever. They hide it in the back of toilets, the base of chairs, the back of speakers, so that even if you nick the main guy, the runners are there to pick up and supply the rest of the stash.

I was calling a taxi one night after a party, at around three o'clock in the morning, and a guy pulls a gun to the back of my head. He gives it, 'I'm a crackhead. I couldn't give a fuck, so give us your stuff.' I had to give it to him.

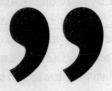

Facts:
Cocaine/crack

Cocaine

'Cocaine is God's way of telling you that you've made too much money.'

(Manager of a rock ' n roll band)

Its history

Chewing coca leaves has been a part of everyday life in South America since at least 2500 BC, but the drug didn't make much impression on Europe until the mid-nineteenth century when German scientists isolated cocaine itself from the coca leaf and used it in patent medicines.

Coca-Cola, containing a few milligrams of cocaine in each glassful, was introduced in 1886 and marketed as an alternative to alcohol. Increasingly, however, cocaine's addictive nature became evident, and in 1903 caffeine replaced cocaine in Coca-Cola. In 1914, the Harrison Act in the US officially outlawed the drug from anything other than medical practice.

Cocaine, as an illegal drug, made a comeback in the mid-1960s and by 1986 it was estimated that 40 per cent of 23–25-year-old North Americans had tried the drug. Its social impact was greatly increased by the appearance of smokable cocaine (crack) in 1985.

Its names

COKE, SNOW, CHARLIE.

Its forms

Cocaine comes in several forms. The one most likely to be encountered in this country is cocaine hydrochloride—a white, crystalline, odourless powder that is soluble in water. It is often mixed with other substances (amphetamines, PCP, or any other white powder that happens to be around) and average purity has recently been put at about 50 per cent. It costs between £50 and £100 per gram.

Cocaine is usually sniffed (snorted) and is sometimes injected, but injecting is dangerous because you never know what the cocaine has been mixed with. The average line of 'coke' usually delivers about 25 milligrams of actual cocaine.

The effects

The effects of cocaine are similar to those of amphetamines. A sense of well-being is produced within minutes and gradually increases. Your confidence grows, as well as your optimism, enthusiasm, and energy. Your self-esteem and your sex-drive improve, and there is an overall feeling of exhilaration and happiness. Most normal pleasures are heightened and there is less need for food, rest, and sleep.

These effects last, however, for minutes rather than hours, and the more you take the drug, the less you feel its effects.

A survey has shown that of cocaine users:

29 per cent take the drug opportunistically

29 per cent take it in a controlled, infrequent way

28 per cent take it more frequently and regularly

14 per cent are compulsive addicts.

Some injecters combine cocaine and heroin in the same syringe (a 'speedball').

The bad effects

Cocaine can increase blood pressure to the point where a stroke occurs, and can cause fits. Too much sniffing can damage the lining of the nose. Pregnant women should avoid it

Excessive doses are likely to produce anxiety and agitation, sweating, dizziness, a high body temperature, a dry mouth, trembling hands and ringing ears. Long-term use can irreversibly damage nerves and small blood vessels in the brain. Heavy doses can cause hallucinations and delusions.

The comedown can be very unpleasant. Users feel hungry, tired, bad tempered and very low. Cocaine is highly addictive, and withdrawal can produce prolonged depression.

The law

Cocaine is a class A drug. You can get up to 7 years for possession and a life sentence for supplying.

Crack

Its names

Crack is also known as PEBBLES, SCUD, WASH, STONE, and ROCK, and it got its original name of 'crack' because of the popping and clicking given off by exploding impurities during smoking.

Its form

Crack is ready-to-use 'freebase' cocaine, which can be smoked in an ordinary pipe, or heated on tin foil and the fumes inhaled. The cocaine is treated with chemicals to free the cocaine base from the hydrochloride.

Crack takes the form of soapy crystals known as rocks or chips and is sold for about £25 for a rock containing a quarter of a gram of freebase cocaine.

The effects

Smoking cocaine this way delivers the drug to the brain at least as rapidly as would be achieved by injection. From the lungs, it goes directly to the brain within seconds, producing an extreme 'rush' and an intense high. People using the drug often fail to find suitable words to describe it, but it is said to be like 'a thousand simultaneous orgasms'.

The high lasts just ten minutes or so, and may be followed by a rapid downswing in mood. Users are left feeling tired, depressed and hungry, and over-sensitive to light and noise. Repeated use leads to the need for larger and larger doses.

Regular smokers often feel irritated and 'wired' and may take heroin to ease the comedown. Bens or alcohol are also used to ease the rough edges of the crack comedown.

The bad effects

Crack smoking is extremely damaging to the lungs and is associated with severe chest pains, bronchitis, and asthma. Pregnant women run the additional risk of giving birth to 'crack babies', who show withdrawal symptoms in the days after birth.

Because of the intense, immediate rush, crack is exceedingly addictive, especially among people who don't feel too good about themselves. Users risk all the unwanted effects listed above under 'Cocaine'.

The law

Like cocaine, crack is a class A drug.

The dealing scene

The final customer in the chain (a girl, 16) . . .

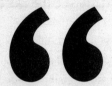

I reckon, at my school, girls and boys deal about equally, though it depends on what you mean by 'dealing'. It's more like a food chain. If I want something, the first people I go to are girls. I know them to say 'Hi' to, and it avoids the 'boy, girl' thing, but I don't see them as dealers. People get these images from films about a criminal element, and it may be like that with hard drugs. With grass and stuff, it's more like someone will say, 'I need a couple of spliffs for a party', and their friend will say, 'OK, give us a tenner. Here's six.' It's like buying fags at a shop.

Take me. I've never bought anything off an original dealer ever. I know who they are. I just have people I know who will buy six spliffs, like I say, and then at a party I can buy a joint off them and pass it around. A bit like sharing a bottle really. You turn up at a party with a bottle of wine, or you turn up with a joint, sort of thing. These friends can offer you grass, but if you want anything more you just tell them and they find it for you. You always know someone who knows someone else.

Actually, most of the kids at my school I get joints off are growing their own at home, but it depends on which one I score off. I have this friend who goes to raves and if she's scoring Es, she'll get some puff for me. I'm sure some stuff is imported—probably from the Netherlands. I reckon in my scene, probably three-quarters of the grass is home grown and a quarter imported.

99

. . . above her, in the London scene (aged 17)

66

The dealers, they're quite criminal. Sorry, but it's true. They're the slug types, and they mug people. The person I score off is a fucking thug—the biggest criminal I've ever met. He's as hard as they come. He mugs other dealers. He's basically a wanker, but he's nice to us because we're regulars. Even the most vicious dealer will cultivate you. He'll take amazing care. What he likes to do is establish himself with a student or, even better, a wealthy 40-year-old who's going to want a large regular supply. What he doesn't want is the geezer who says, 'All right mate, let's have a couple of Es then.' No future in that, is there?

In our age group, we've got 16 and 17-year-old dealers at school and they're not going to sell to 40-year-olds. Our ones are usually trying to get a couple of ounces off at a time. The geezer we get ours off is into quarters. There's a lot of other dealers who do it totally differently though. They've all got different styles and they deal in different amounts. I know six or seven kids at school who are dealing, and they're all completely different too.

You don't even have to have money in London. You can get stuff on tick if you know the dealer. If you're skint, you can go on tick with several dealers—do the rounds. There are horror stories though of going on tick and then not being able to pay it back—people getting their kneecaps broken, or having to work as runners, and not being able to get out. The thing is, with girls having tick— they won't get beaten up. But if us boys go on tick and don't pay back, the dealer will get heavy with us. Our dealer gets quite upset by that. 'The girls, they won't pay me back and there's nothing I can do.' But us—we have to pay back.

I don't know with dealers though. Every now and then your dealer will bring in something 'other' and they'll tell you about it. You can be led on that way. You think, 'Oh well, it's there, so I might as well try it.'

99

The users turned dealers
A 22-year-old

66

For a long time, drugs were very mysterious to me. I had heard people talking about this stuff called marijuana, but my impression was it was an exotic spice. In the early days, when I was too young to score, I used to go into my elder brother's room when he was out and scan his floor with a vacuum cleaner which had a piece of gauze attached to the nozzle. I'd pick up blims which I would then stick down cigarettes to smoke, because I had no idea how to make a joint.

I see drugs now as a good tranquillizer. They stop me getting bored and enable me to drift and dream. I like puff particularly because it allows one to objectify experience. But I was first drawn towards drugs because they weren't allowed and because they were different. I also associated

drugs with insanity and with different levels of conscious-
ness. They are now central to the traveller culture to which I
belong.

Drugs are also the main ritual and the main source of
income, hence most of the travellers' names—Easy-E, Cuts,
Blim and Stacker. Breakfast is when the ritual begins. We
will eat something quickly, pour some coffee, and then skin
up. We probably smoke an eighth each per day.

I have sold hash—initially just to support my own
habit, but later to make money. I think I got a buzz out of
walking around with a big lump of hash in my pocket. It was
a rush, I thought I was Scarface. When I was at university, I
would go round the Union with a big Roses tin, shaking it
and saying, 'Anyone want to buy hash?' I would make a
hundred quid in an evening, and spend thirty on beer.

The most I have ever made in one deal is about
£2,000 on five kilos of hash. That was about three removed
from source, but my brother used to buy it nearly directly
from importation. He told me this story once of someone
smuggling in dope by moulding it into the shape of a brief-
case, painting it, and walking through Customs. I know of a
lot of people who will go to Amsterdam and come back with
four or five ounces in their stomach. I have heard of people
carrying as much as half a kilo in their stomach, covered in
beeswax, but they all have bowel problems now.

In London I briefly started dealing in coke. I got very
arrogant and selfish about this. I thought it was decadent
and flash. There was glamour attached. I used to get
famous people scoring from me, and I developed a cocky
persona.

99

A 24-year-old

"

I started dealing when I was 18 and left school. I found that being on the dole, it was the best way to make money, without having to declare it. When I started buying hash, I soon realized that it would be better to buy more. I could then buy cheap and support myself selling ounces in eighths. I'd have a constant supply to keep me happy, skimming off blims here and there.

To begin with I just sold hash to mates. Then I started buying it in larger amounts until I was buying nine bars (nine ounces), half kilos and then kilos. At this stage I wouldn't sell less than ounces at a time. I suppose in the hierarchy of things, I was now at the next stage—supplying suppliers. It was glamorous—I had a mobile, I had money, and I had reputation.

With this came risk and danger. The harder they come, the harder they fall as it were. But the point is, I'm earning—and more than my mates stacking shelves at Sainsbury's. More than that, there's a buzz to dealing, you feel 'large'. People come to you. Forget this myth that we're desperadoes standing on street corners. This is a demand led market.

In a way, the buzz you get comes from fear of getting nicked, and ultimately everyone's in this to get out. If the law doesn't get to you the paranoia will, and the higher up you go the more serious it all gets. To begin with, it was all fun and games. I used to walk around outside school, dealing with a spliff hanging out of my mouth and an 'Adihash' T-shirt on. I look back now and think I was a fucking fool. But I had less to lose then.

Nowadays, things are strictly business. If I didn't treat it like that it would be my downfall. I've had too many crusty mates taken by the pigs because they're walking round like it's the summer of '69. The advantage of being bigger is economies of scale, and my profits are larger. But it also means I'm handling less people directly and can keep the whole business more discreet. Ultimately you don't know who your enemies are, and who's watching and listening. But I can't get too paranoid or I'll lose my marbles.

If you worry too much, you make your fears come true, like a mate of mine who was dealing and had to go into the mental ward because he thought police helicopters were watching him wherever he went. After a while, every time he was set to make a big deal, he'd have to check his oracle and the stars. He was wandering into the realms of fantasy, and do you know why? Because he was consuming too much of what he was selling.

Rule One: if you want to make money, and don't want to get nicked, don't bosh what you're selling.

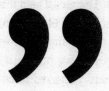

Facts:
Heroin

Its history

Heroin belongs to a group of drugs called opiates, made from the opium poppy. Opium provided comfort for the Egyptians, the Greeks, the Persians, and the Romans. In the nineteenth century its use was widespread in Britain and many other countries, and writers like Thomas de Quincey, Samuel Coleridge, Wilkie Collins, and Charles Dickens all took opium. The drug was cheap and easily available and familiar to all levels of society.

Opium-containing medicines were widely used for calming children, and the resulting mortality gave cause for concern. The introduction of the Pharmacy Act in 1868 restricted the sale of opium to registered chemists, and after the First World War non-medical use of opiates was forbidden. The widespread use of heroin emerged again in the 1960s, followed by large-scale importation of black market heroin.

Its names

Heroin is also known as SMACK, JUNK, GEAR, BROWN or SKAG.

Its form

Pure diamorphine is a white powder, but street heroin is brownish in colour. It can be injected, sniffed or smoked. For smoking, the drug is placed on some tin foil and heated. The fumes are then inhaled through another piece of foil rolled into a tube, a method sometimes known as 'chasing the dragon'. On the streets, heroin will be cut with other substances such as glucose, and sold as £10 or £20 'bags' or 'wraps'.

The purity of street heroin ranges widely from 10 to 80 per cent, and present prices are quite static at about £80 per gram. Street heroin reaches the user through a massive network of pyramid selling. The importer has a number of distributors who connect with people who buy a few pounds of heroin in weight. They in turn sell to others in ounces, and these ounce dealers are often users themselves. The next level consists of street users who buy a few grams at a time and parcel these out in smaller quantities. The drug becomes more adulterated at every stage of this journey.

The effects

Heroin creates a sense of psychic warmth and well-being in which pain and anxiety disappear. It can make your skin feel itchy and you may nod off and wake up several times. For the first-time user there can be immediate and unpleasant side-effects like nausea and vomiting.

The bad effects

Surveys suggest that people who experiment with heroin or other opiates run a very high risk of becoming both physically and mentally dependent, and there are very real risks of overdose, infection and serious accident. Damage to the body is common, caused by repeated injections with dirty needles and by the substances that are often mixed with the drug. The chances of dying are even greater if other drugs, such as alcohol, are used at the same time.

Regular heroin users are often in poor health because of an inadequate diet. They suffer from constipation and in women the menstrual cycle is often interrupted.

Withdrawal or 'clucking' can be very unpleasant, with increasing anxiety, restlessness, and irritability. You start to yawn, stretch, and sweat, and your eyes and nose begin to stream, with frequent sneezing. You then get nausea and pains in your stomach, often with uncontrollable diarrhoea. Trembling, aching in the bones and muscles, terror and insomnia complete the picture. Your skin is pale and clammy, and covered in goose bumps (hence the term 'cold turkey'). Your legs twitch and thrash ('kicking the habit'). These symptoms are at their height for two or three days and then gradually subside over the next couple of weeks. The life of most addicts is organized around ensuring that 'clucking' never happens.

The law

Heroin is a class A drug. You can get up to 7 years for possession and life imprisonment for supplying.

Chief Inspector Andy Smith

has been in the police force for twenty-six years, most of which time has been spent in North London. He is now a Community Liaison Officer for Barnet and Hertsmere with special responsibility for linking with other services, especially over drugs—training in drugs awareness, drugs education, and dealing with persistent young offenders.

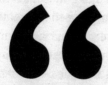

WHAT IS THE PROBLEM?

When I got here, two and a half years ago, I was told, 'There is no drug problem here.' The fact is that was rubbish and we just had our heads in the sand. I've distilled my job down to five main areas of activity—drugs, bullying, truancy, racism, and domestic violence. But I'm mainly dealing with drugs, not because it is flavour of the month, but because it's become a real issue. We've set up a drug forum which aims to co-ordinate the response to issues to do with young people and substance abuse in the local area. There was a lot going on but not enough co-operation. We needed to start working together, and the government White Paper *Tackling Drugs Together* has confirmed this as the way forward.

We all have the same job—to raise young people's awareness about drugs so that they can make informed decisions. I'm quite comfortable with that approach, and I don't mind sitting on the same platform as someone promoting the legalization of drugs because I think debate is good. Personally, I don't agree with legalization but there are arguments on both sides. We all need to listen to one another's evidence, particularly over the harm cannabis can cause. We need to be aware of all the issues.

WHY DO YOUNG PEOPLE USE DRUGS?

There are probably the same number of reasons as for any other human behaviour. There are hundreds of reasons why people use alcohol, and the same applies to other drugs. It's a thrill, it's nice, it's something they need to do—you can go on endlessly; but each case that becomes a crisis has to be looked at in a totally individual way. We have to be sensitive enough to respond differently and to try to understand the different circumstances each time.

The use of cannabis is undoubtedly widespread—not only in schools, but in homes and clubs—and therefore tolerance by the public is alarmingly high. This may be a refusal to acknowledge it's happening, or a lack of knowledge, or maybe people simply don't mind the use of drugs in their homes. But they have to realize that although cannabis is not technically addictive, some people can become dependent on it.

HOW CAN YOU HELP PARENTS AND TEACHERS?

It's not just young people we have to help. We have to raise parents' awareness, because there are often things being done and said at home that parents don't tune into. Teachers also need to have their awareness raised and a 'whole school' approach is what we are promoting.

Basically we are saying, 'It's all very well going into the classroom and giving young people information but it's got to be reinforced in the staffroom so that teachers are confident about tackling the issues. Parents need to be informed as well, so that they can carry on the discussion.'

The amount of ignorance is appalling. I've been to school meetings of parents, governors and teachers where they don't even understand obvious expressions like 'spliffs'. I have to refer to them as 'joints'. They've heard about speed but don't know what it is, or what an ecstasy tablet looks like, or what it can do to you.

WHAT ARE THE SIGNS THAT SOMEONE IS USING DRUGS?

When I'm asked that by parents I say, 'Well, I can tell you but they can also be attributed to thirty or forty other things—like having a headache, or a period, or whatever.' I say, 'Don't jump to conclusions.' Then they ask, 'What does the paraphernalia look like?' 'Well,' I reply, 'Silver foil—but that is just as likely to mean that your son is eating chocolate in bed!'

Some parents are really panicking and the danger is that they will over-react and push their offspring even further away. I don't condone or encourage the use of drugs in any shape or form, but it is a fact of life that a few young people will use drugs heavily and then it becomes a very real issue. However, the statistics show that if young people do try drugs, mostly it's just experimental. They try them once or twice and then move on to something else. They don't get hooked on drugs.

I tell parents that just because you smoke one spliff, it doesn't mean you're going to become a heroin addict. But I do add that all the heroin addicts I know started on spliffs and speed. I tell them about the 'gateway theory'—that you don't just go straight into heroin. You go through a process of initiation into the drug culture. I also point out that 110,000 people each year die from tobacco related diseases in this country, and another 60,000 die as a result of alcohol. These are by far the most dangerous drugs we've got and the most widely used. They are both drugs, and glue is a drug, and they are all legally available. We can't just say we'll deal with narcotics. We've got to deal with the whole package—all drugs that alter your personality and the way you work.

When I go into schools to talk to parents and teachers, I tell them it's not just cannabis, speed, and coke they should be worrying about, but also alcohol and tobacco. If we can prevent young people from smoking and drinking at an early age, then maybe we can prevent a lot more people trying other substances. I wish more money could be spent on research into cannabis use—like the possibility that it may stay around in your body for up to a month as the breakdown substances get taken up in the fatty tissues in your body; and when you're driving on Monday or Tuesday, you may still be under the effects of a spliff smoked the Saturday before.

WHAT IS THE ROLE OF THE POLICE?

There is a school of thought in the police force that we are only an enforcement agency, but I take a different stance and believe we are also concerned with prevention. We should take a two-fold approach to drugs and deal with supply and demand. We've been dealing with supply for years, mainly unsuccessfully. From available evidence, we are probably only getting hold of about 10 per cent of what's floating about. If we could deal with the demand side as well, we would have a much more positive effect on the whole scene.

Locally, we've adopted a policy whereby we are not looking to put people into the criminal justice system. We are aiming instead at early intervention—when kids are only just getting into drugs. If we march in and say, 'Right, you're nicked, down the station,' that just polarizes the situation. The young person simply gets alienated from society. Our role is certainly not frightening people—shock horror tactics are old hat. What we've got to do is help the casual user make informed decisions. We use ex-drug users who are extraordinarily effective at talking to young people. They don't dress it up, but sell it as it is: the awful processes they've gone through, the low self-esteem, the resorting to prostitution, and what it's like to come off.

And locally, nationally and internationally we must carry on tracking down the dealers and stopping the drugs coming on to the market. I am aware that whole nations survive on their drug economies, but I can't make allowances for that.

HOW SHOULD PARENTS DEAL WITH CHILDREN OVER THE DRUG SCENE?

I think that first they've got to rationalize their own position over the use of other substances. Dad drinks, Mum smokes, they both take pills every day of the week. How they deal with that when talking to their kids depends on their own skills and their ability to communicate. You can't ignore smoking and drinking, you can't say to your child, 'You can't do cannabis, but it's OK if we smoke and drink.' It's just not logical and young people pick that up instantly.

The next thing parents should do, and we may be able to help here, is brush up on their knowledge of drugs, so that they know what to do if there is any suspicion, or if the child is actually found with drugs. The best advice is, 'Don't panic.'

WHAT ATTITUDE SHOULD SCHOOLS HAVE?

Expulsion from school is a big issue, and we try to work with schools over that. We say, 'Let's deal with this problem together.' I think someone who uses should be given another chance. We've all heard stories about young people who've been using being expelled from school when taking examinations and who subsequently commit suicide. Surely that must not be allowed to happen? There may come a time, if children in school are dealing, when expulsion does become essential. My personal view is that schools should take a rigorous stance over the use of all substances, so that it is very clear what the rules are, but not be so inflexible that, no matter what the circumstances, the pupil gets chucked out. It has to be made clear that drinking and smoking will not be tolerated either. Do the staff smoke? Is there a 'no smoking' policy throughout the school? Why should it be all right to go into the staffroom and be choked by nicotine? This gives very mixed messages.

I do need to make the point here that there is no evidence that drugs are more likely to be used by any particular group of young people, say, from one ethnic group or another. That is a load of tripe. Drug taking is right across the board and, while we are on the subject, most people who get arrested for drugs are white. The problem is classless, raceless and genderless — or rather, it's equal among both sexes.

WHAT ARE THE POWERS OF AN ARRESTING OFFICER?

The procedure that young people will come up against can vary from one police officer to another, but the basic script is something like this. The police officer sees someone whom he or she suspects is in possession of drugs. The officer has the right of search under the Misuse of Drugs Act and can, to a certain extent, search someone there and then in the street. If the officer suspects that a more intimate search might be required, the suspect will be taken to a private place or to the police station.

The officer has the power to arrest the suspect in the street. There is then a series of different things that might happen — depending on the gravity of the situation. Each case is assessed individually and each case has a 'disposal option' of between one and five, one being the least severe. Suppose it's a case of assault. The option then is four, which means the person is more likely to be charged. The *Case Disposal Manual* that we follow is used service wide, so the way we deal with a drugs case here would not be dissimilar to the way it would be dealt with anywhere else.

HOW SHOULD PARENTS BEHAVE WHEN THEIR CHILD GETS BUSTED?

Not many young people get taken down to the police station for drugs, but they obviously do occasionally. The parent needs to act like an enlightened parent—supportive, attentive, questioning why it has happened. Shouting and screaming, or walking into the custody suite and clipping the child round the ear, certainly does not help. This might make the parent feel better for thirty seconds but the child feels even further away. I think parents should try to use the event as an opportunity to stop the situation developing, and ask us and anyone else they can think of to help. There are a lot of different agencies.

Being hostile to the police does not help. If parents think there has been a breach in the criminal justice system, they are entitled to question it and I would encourage them to do so. They can then seek the appropriate legal advice.

WHAT ARE THE CHILD'S RIGHTS?

Up to the age of 17, if children are brought into the police station for questioning, for processes like fingerprint taking or having their rights read to them, or for being formally charged or bailed, they must be accompanied by a parent or guardian. If these are not available our codes of practice say we have to call out a member of the social services to act in *loco parentis*. If the social services are not available, there is a group of people referred to as 'appropriate adults'.

We have set up a panel of people who can be called out on a twenty-four hour basis, and act as an enlightened parent would act to make sure that the rights of the young person are respected. They make sure that there is no ambiguity in the questions asked, that the young person understands what's going on, and that his or her welfare is being considered. They can stop the interview at any stage, and they can call in a solicitor at any time.

The rights of silence need to be observed; and not just observed but explained to parents, because of the consequences nowadays of remaining silent.

WHAT ARE THE ALTERNATIVES IF YOU ARE ARRESTED FOR DRUG POSSESSION?

If you are a juvenile, there are several different ways you may be handled. If you are charged, you will be dealt with in a Youth Court and if you are convicted, that conviction will be with you for as long as the offence remains on record, in accordance with the Rehabilitation of Offenders Act.

You may instead receive a formal caution under which you are told, basically, that you have been arrested for an offence. You have to admit to the offence and say that you are willing to receive a caution. This will go on a police record which is not the same as a criminal record. Once you reach the age of 17, provided that you haven't been in trouble with the police again, the police record is destroyed and can never be used against you in court. Cautions can be quoted against you in court until you are 17.

Another alternative is a formal warning, which is slightly different. This does not require the consent of the person, nor do they have to admit that they have carried out the offence, but there has to be credible evidence that they are guilty. As the police are not proceeding further though, there is only a local record of the offence.

WHAT ARE THE CONSEQUENCES OF HAVING A CRIMINAL RECORD?

Having a criminal record does you no good at all. It can result, for instance, in visas being refused for travel to certain countries. When you apply for jobs, there are certain professions—teaching, the police, working in the National Health Service—where you've got to declare that you have a criminal record. You do have the right, after a certain period of time, under the Rehabilitation of Offenders Act, to say you have no criminal convictions, even if you've had one in the past; but up to that time, which is specified in the Act, you do have to declare it.

Having a criminal record doesn't necessarily mean that you won't get a job. You can even join the police force with a criminal record. But it might make the difference between you getting the job and someone else getting it. Jobs are difficult enough to come by without having a criminal record.

It is also not good for the offender's family, or for the offender's self-esteem. Generally speaking, the longer you can remain without a conviction—even a driving conviction—the better it is for you as an individual. If, for instance, you get arrested and convicted for driving under the influence of drugs, there are insurance consequences and your driver's licence will be taken away. These are all things which young people need to be told about.

HOW CAN THE POLICE TELL
IF SOMEONE HAS BEEN SMOKING CANNABIS?

A lot of young people think that because we can't smell cannabis on their breath, they won't get caught. But there is a blood test we can do and if we suspect drugs, we take a blood specimen. For instance, if you are seen to be driving in such a manner that the police suspect you are under the influence of alcohol or drugs, and you breathalyse negative, the police have the right to take you to the police station. They will then ask to take a blood sample. Unlike alcohol, there is no precise limit on drugs. If you have drugs in your bloodstream, that's it.

WHAT ABOUT DECRIMINALIZATION?

I've looked at all the arguments and I've found none that persuade me that legalization or decriminalization is the right course of action. There is a debate still going on in Holland about whether to legalize drugs; and there are many people in Holland who think that even decriminalization has been a disaster. We have enough substances legalized—tobacco, alcohol—without adding to them. Personally, I don't think legalization would reduce crime. It would reduce the number of people arrested for possession or supplying, but many of the problems we deal with are due to the way people behave when under the influence of drugs.

SHOULD THERE BE MORE POWERS FOR THE POLICE OVER DRUGS?

I don't think we need more powers. I think the criminal law as we have it is fine. What we need is more resources. I would like extra staff to go into schools, I would like training packages, I would like the resources to implement the government's policies in *Tackling Drugs Together*. I would like to see even more co-operation between the various services concerned.

Drugs is an issue, so let's deal with it before it becomes worse. We are not waging war against drugs—they're inanimate objects. What we are trying to do is work together with young people—those that use drugs and those that don't, and especially the vulnerable ones.

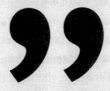

Facts:

The law

Some definitions:

A Juvenile

At 17 years or below you are a juvenile. When you make a statement, or are given a caution, a parent or guardian, or someone acting in *loco parentis* (which means 'in the place of a parent') must be present. A juvenile offender can also request the presence of a solicitor. (See also the Facts section 'If you get arrested', pp. 52–4.)

The Case Disposal System

This system, which is outlined in the *Case Disposal Manual*, helps the police to decide what action to take. In an attempt to achieve consistency throughout the country over how cases are dealt with, the manual contains a list of common offences, each with a case disposal option number and a list of aggravating and mitigating circumstances relating to the offence. A section of the manual called 'The General Gravity Factor Section' guides the police on how to take an appropriate course of action. They have four alternatives in dealing with an offender:

(1)   to proceed with a prosecution
(2)   to give a formal caution
(3)   to give a formal warning
(4)   not to proceed with a prosecution.

Each case is decided on its own merits.

Prosecution

In the case of juvenile crime, the police try to avoid this course of action. However, it is as well to know that under the terms of the Misuse of Drugs Act (1971) you are more likely to go to court if you are caught with a class A drug, however small the quantity; and, in general, sentences for supply or trafficking are enforced more rigorously than those of possession.

Cautioning of Offenders

The purpose of a formal caution is to deal quickly and simply with less serious offenders, preserving them from any unnecessary appearance in the criminal courts and reducing the chances of them re-offending.

The national standards for cautioning are:

- there must be sufficient evidence of the offender's guilt to make the prospect of prosecution realistic
- the offender (and in the case of a juvenile, the parent or guardian too) must understand the significance of a caution and must consent to the caution being given.

The offender is informed that:

- a central record of the offence will be kept
- the caution may be cited in court if the offender is subsequently found guilty of another offence.

Formal Warning of Offenders

Formal warnings are used instead of cautions for minor or trivial offences.

Offenders are told that:

- a local record will be kept for three years

——————— a previous warning may influence the decision whether or not to prosecute if the person re-offends

——————— a formal warning cannot be cited in court.

No Prosecution

In the past, many offences were classified as 'No Further Action' where there was clear evidence of a person's guilt but for various reasons it was decided not to proceed. A new category of case disposal, 'Not Proceeded With', has now been introduced to enable such offences to be treated as a crime solved.

Decriminalization

The act of drug possession or use of a drug remains illegal but the law is not enforced.

John is a drug counsellor

at a drug rehabilitation centre in South London. He's been working in drug centres for eight years and thinks that the drug scene at the worst end will get worse and the clientele younger.

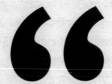

Almost everyone we see is under 20. The youngest we have had to counsel is a 7-year-old, and we have also had a number of 8 and 9-year-olds, but the bulk of our clientele are 12 to 16. I do a lot of work in primary schools. I will talk to 8-year-olds and, on average, between a third and a half will debate with you whether a three or a five-skin joint is better!

It sounds odd to say this but the major problem drug among young people is cannabis, especially the super-skunk coming in now. Everyone says it's 'not a big deal', but people will travel miles at three in the morning with all their money to get some! We have a lot of kids who get into debt problems over it. Say you get ten quid pocket money and you buy an eighth. You are a fiver short. The dealers will sub you for that, but your debt builds up. In the end they call in the debt, and if you haven't got it you're in the shit. Your choices are you go out nicking or into prostitution. If you can't do that, you end up working for one of them, and then it begins to get seriously nasty.

I had one kid who ended up shifting cocaine for a crack group. When he was 15 he decided he wanted out. These people took him down to a cellar where there was this guy tied up naked. They pasted him with sugar and water with a wallpaper brush and then peeled it off. Of course, all his skin came off too. They said, 'This is what happens to people who want out. How serious are you about leaving?' The kid comes to us and says he wants a safe house. He's ducking and diving and can't stay at one address for any length of time, and there are shotguns pointed at him from car windows. It's completely nuts.

E is a problem, but I say E in a broad sense. We get a lot analysed, and the last six had no E in them. They had K (ketamine) and caffeine, K and orphenadine, K and selegiline (the treatment for Parkinson's disease). Ketamine is legal so the only thing the police can get the dealers on is fraud! The psychological effects of these Es has been very damaging. We had a lot of kids come in mid-week who have become psychotic. The other day, a normally very relaxed boy for no apparent reason hammered his mother over the smallest of disagreements.

The way we deal with it is in the open. Why should we drive it underground? They won't legalize it, though that would be the sane response. As one government minister said to me, 'It's not even up for discussion.' They don't want to deal with the problem. It's the biggest business in the world, the banks would collapse, and we'd have a revolution. They want it contained but not dealt with.

Here we try to deliver information in a credible way. It's no good having the police chat to kids because no one believes them. It's no good having teachers try and sort it out because they still talk about 'pot'! So what we do is train up young people who have been there, seen it, done it, and let them take over.

The up and coming problem is crack, which until recently had only affected the 18s and over. Now it is filtering down to the younger kids. We are working with 12-year-olds at present. We have 14 to 15-year-olds spending £700 a week on it, obtained by prostitution, drug running, car thefts. There is some gross stuff going on. We've worked out that the average sum spent by a crack user is £1,500 a week. But five-figure numbers are not unusual. I know one guy who got through £26,000 in a fortnight.

I had a call from the local hospital the other day, saying, 'We have one of your clients here.' I go down and the doctor says, 'Is 17 grams of coke in an hour a lethal dose?' I mean, he's asking me? Meanwhile my client's sitting bolt upright in his bed saying, 'We ought to get out of here now.' So I'm saying, 'Relax, relax.' Next thing, he's off down the corridor at 100 miles per hour, with me behind him saying, 'What's going on?' He says, 'I've got to get to the car,' and then, in a whisper, 'It's full of coke.' I had to drive him to the dealer and sell back the coke just to keep him from killing himself, he was so far gone and, believe me, it was no small amount. And this scene is not unusual.

In the North, it tends to be more sedatives, like heroin. The received impression is that the crack scene is mainly black, but it isn't, it's just that the black scene is more overt. The white crack scene is more underground, and tends to be in people's houses rather than on the street. Drugs are across the board—they give equal opportunities!

The music scene is a big focus for drugs. Jungle music, for example, which is very big around here, goes hand in hand with coke. The drugs now control the music unlike before when it was the other way around. For example, three years ago it was all happy House music because that went with the good Es around then. Quite often, the dealers control the music that is played at raves or clubs, because they are the ones with the money. They organize the music that goes best with the drugs they want to promote. The two are inextricably linked.

GBH is big at the moment. We had some girls last year who'd been given it and told to inject it by some blokes obviously looking for sex. It's fifteen quid a cap and it's legal—it's usually mixed with caustic soda and solvents. The effects depend on how you mix it up, and are anything from feeling as randy as shit (you would screw anything that moved, you don't even have to move, you would make love to this desk) to your legs and arms shaking uncontrollably, or respiratory arrest, or nothing at all. It's completely random and depends on the batch.

We've had a lot of ketamine victims but that is largely through kak Es. Some of them end up rigid with lockjaw, staying in the same position for hours and unable to talk. We have quite a lot of acid in the area. It used to be about 90 micrograms in strength, but now microdots are coming back that are about 160. That's hallucination strength.

Nowadays there's a different scene associated with drugs. It's not so much sitting around with joss-sticks expanding the mind. It's more wandering around the town, playing computer games and going to the arcade. The main difference between then and now is that there isn't any 'love and peace' malarkey. Today we buy love and peace and swallow it down on a Saturday night, and come back to reality on Monday. That about sums it up.

One has to remember Newton's law—every action has an equal and opposite reaction. So although it's all comrades on Saturday night, come Wednesday when everyone's clucking, you have a very volatile situation. More than that, people can't deal with being up and down all the time, it's schizophrenic. People come to us and they genuinely can't recognize good from bad any more.

In tackling all this, one has to remember that, by and large, at the time, drugs are just so bloody nice. One can't deny the initial appeal of them, otherwise people wouldn't take them. That's why the heroin campaigns never worked. They were a lie. People would think, 'If it's so bloody awful, why do all my mates take it and have a good time?' I mean, ask any crackhead what their first lick was like and they will tell you 'God-like.' We can't deny the appeal when we are dealing with the drug problem or we lose all credibility.

Around here, it doesn't take much to realize why they start either. Out of 165 school leavers last year at the local school, two got jobs after six months. In such an environment, you don't have to do much promoting as a dealer to make your drugs tempting. It's just a cheap mental breakout from a very depressing situation. There are a lot of people out there kicking around with nothing to do. What are you going to do about it? Drugs are the perfect answer—artificial fun. 'Let's do some now.'

This is the perfect environment for dealers. They're everywhere. Within ten seconds of walking out of this building, you could score anything. Dealing's the only job you can get around here. The kids think, 'Why should I consider myself lucky to work for £2 an hour stacking shelves in the corner shop when my mate's selling crack and driving a BMW?'

In a way, it's a sane response to an insane situation. But the image of pushers on street corners shoving drugs at you is rubbish. Let's make no mistake, this is a sellers' market. It is demand led. People come to them, it isn't door-to-door sales. This idea of peer pressure is crap as well— peer temptation maybe. If it is all around you, before long you look at it and say, 'I'll have some of that.' People opt in. It is a user-friendly culture. I've never seen anyone say, 'Oi, take this—or else.' That's an adult misconception.

But I've never seen the level of heaviness that's about now. Everyone's got guns and is tooled up to the teeth. If you talk to most of the kids out here, they could tell you where to get a gun. We've had several gunfights—passing cars just popping off at each other across the street.

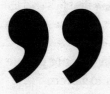

Dr Philip Robson is a consultant psychiatrist

who works in a drug dependency unit in Oxford and specializes in helping people with drug problems from alcohol through to heroin.

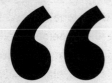

**IS DRUG TAKING A REAL PROBLEM
OR SOMETHING IN SOCIETY WE JUST HAVE TO ACCEPT?**

There are certainly problems we have to face up to, even with the experimental use of drugs. First, there is the reaction to it by parents and teachers—itself a tremendous problem. I heard recently of someone being thrown out of a school near Oxford for smoking cannabis just before A levels. Now how is that going to help him, his parents, or anyone else?

The second problem is the drug taking itself. All drug taking carries risks. The risks with some drugs may have been exaggerated and people may be emphasizing the wrong risks for the wrong drugs. But there is no such thing as a 'risk-free drug': there are short and long-term risks. The people who take those risks have to weigh them up against the benefits, and not distort the facts in order to convince themselves that there are no risks.

But drug use, or rather drug abuse, is usually a symptom of something else being wrong rather than simply a problem in itself. As with alcohol, the vast majority of young drug users are taking them experimentally and are able to moderate their use so that it does not become a problem.

Research was undertaken in America, where they followed 100 children from 3 to 18, including interviews with their parents, in which, among other things, they looked at drug taking behaviour. As the children grew older, their psychological profiles suggested that the experimental users of drugs were the healthy group, and the abstainers from experimentation were 'relatively tense, over controlled, emotionally restricted individuals who were somewhat socially isolated and lacking in interpersonal skills'. The heavy users of drugs tended to be 'troubled adolescents who were interpersonally alienated, emotionally withdrawn, and manifestly unhappy, who expressed their maladjustment through under controlled and overtly antisocial behaviour'.

This gives rise to the difficult concept, particularly for parents, that if their children are going to become leaders, then they may well be the kind of people who experiment with life, and that, as I've pointed out, carries increased risks. But remember that work, sex, food, and gambling can all be experimented with as well, and can also lead to addictive patterns of behaviour. They too have their problems and risks.

So are all the answers to do with education about drugs?

If you look at the research on this, effective education isn't just about giving the facts. Learning about drugs doesn't necessarily alter behaviour, any more than it does with smoking. You have to involve young people themselves in discussions—information exchange rather than information overload. Most teachers haven't used drugs themselves, so they've got as much to learn from young people as they have to teach.

Another lesson that is needed is to help young people develop necessary skills. If they don't particularly want to smoke or take drugs, but all their friends are doing it, they need the social skills to say 'no' but keep their friends. This is the additional component of a successful school prevention programme.

There is suggestive evidence from further research in America that the combination of giving information and social skills training does alter behaviour. This is certainly the best way forward that we have at the moment.

The information given about the risks of drug taking must be relevant to the particular person at that particular time. For instance, if young people are smoking cannabis, emphasizing that it may give them bronchitis in twenty years' time is not helpful. It won't have an effect because the danger is too remote. The short-term pleasure will trump the long-term risk every time. Being informed that smoking cannabis may affect your A level results next week has more immediacy and will have much more effect.

It is more effective to present information about drugs in discussion rather than in a lecture—and this applies as much to parents as to teachers. If young people are involved in discussion, they can bring up important points. One of the most famous sayings of Tim Beck, an originator of 'cognitive' therapy, is: 'I believe what I hear myself say.' It is much more valuable if someone comes to a conclusion and states it himself than has someone else tell him what is right.

AT WHAT AGE DO YOU THINK WE SHOULD START
TO DISCUSS DRUGS WITH YOUNG PEOPLE?

There appear to be two tasks here. We need to delay drug taking by people who haven't already started—and that applies as much to smoking and alcohol as it does to illegal drugs. For this you need to be looking at the under-12s because most of the research shows that by the age of 13 children are getting into the initiation stage, which requires a different approach. If you direct education programmes aimed at children who haven't yet tried a drug at those who are using them, it can be counter-productive. They may 'catastrophize' drugs and think, 'Well, if it's that bad and I've gone this far, I might as well go the whole hog.'

Another thing that research shows is that the younger you get into both legal (tobacco and alcohol) and illegal drugs—and I wouldn't want to separate those two—the more risk there is of problems later on. With younger children you need to be specific and spell out the facts in black and white, because boundaries are appreciated by the young; but you should still be encouraging discussion, not offering horror stories or exaggeration.

The other group is the 'harm reduction' group—13-plus—who, if not actually using drugs themselves, will almost certainly know someone who is. They will have had some first-hand exposure to drugs and will want clear information, and advice perhaps on how to say 'no'. You should also be encouraging those who are using to do so in a safe and sensible way.

Generally, harm reduction should be based around the cliché 'Using the drug and not having the drug use you,' but the vast majority of young people who get into drugs are just flirting with them. It's no big deal, and again it is important that the drugs education should not turn it into one.

WHAT FACTORS LEAD THE EXPERIMENTER TO BECOME A SOCIAL USER AND THE SOCIAL USER TO BECOME A COMPULSIVE ONE?

The reason why people become compulsive users seems to depend on three characteristics. The first is the individual personality. The second is the social environment. Experimentation is across all social classes, but at the compulsive user end there are many more people from poor and socially deprived backgrounds. The third is the pharmacology of the drug being used. Some drugs are much more likely to lead to addiction, and the purity of the drug, the dose, and the route by which it is taken are all very important. It is wrong, therefore, to see it in simply chemical terms, with crack and heroin being regarded as incredibly addictive. Yes, they do have the right pharmacology in that they make you feel very pleasant, but in order for you to become addicted, there have to be other things going on at the same time.

However, if you take the end point of addiction—helpless or compulsive drug taking—I see people from totally normal backgrounds with quite robust personalities who have become addicted. Here we have to raise the possibility that there is some biological element missing which the drug has replaced. I also see people from deprived backgrounds who have had no chance in life. Drugs offer them a way of life and a temporary niche. A classic junkie has membership of a club—a way of behaving, with rules, a way of life.

WHAT ARE THE MOST COMMON PROBLEMS YOU ARE SEEING IN YOUR UNIT?

You have to realize that people come to us only if there is a major problem. Many people with drug problems turn first to parents, friends, self-help groups or family doctors. So what we are seeing and treating in the unit does not tell us much about the nature of illegal drug taking going on in the community as a whole.

Something like a third of the people we see are under 25, and not infrequently under 17. In more than 70 per cent of cases, they are on heroin or other opiates. The second most common drug is amphetamine. It is harder to treat many amphetamine users because of the nature of the drug and the way it is taken. We don't often see ecstasy users, but about one in ten has a primary problem with cannabis.

A lot of people we see who have drug related problems are not actually addicted in the sense of being physically or psychologically dependent. Their problems can be physical or psychological, or they may have social or legal difficulties. What we offer is 'listening', and beyond that we try to provide what each individual needs. This may be some kind of psychological support—individually or in a group; a substitute drug, or some other pharmacological intervention.

If people are addicted, there are two stages to the treatment. Detoxification is the act of getting off the regular use of the drug. This in itself isn't effective unless it is linked to something beyond. The addict has to break the previous patterns of his or her life. This may mean moving away to live somewhere new, or starting a new relationship; or it might mean going into a rehabilitation programme.

The research which indicates what the best treatments are, and whether what we are doing is successful, is very limited. This is because the research is difficult to do. Drug taking is, after all, an illegal activity.

WHAT DO YOU CONSIDER THE MOST DANGEROUS DRUGS AROUND?

That is almost impossible to answer. Ecstasy, for instance, can have an unpredictable and idiosyncratic effect which can knacker you completely, but this is incredibly rare. It's like playing Russian roulette with several thousand chambers! It's not worth it for me, but it might be for someone of a different age, with a different life-style. It is a cost-benefit analysis each time.

Crack is potentially one of the most dangerous drugs; but if you take into account how widespread the use is of different drugs, then you have to come down to tobacco. This is second only to alcohol in prevalence of use, is the most highly addictive, and has the worst outcome per user.

Another way of looking at this question is to ask about acute reactions. According to Emergency Room statistics from the US, cocaine produces the most admissions. However, from an adolescent's point of view, I would rate cannabis as the riskiest drug. It is by far the most commonly used illegal drug and because it is illegal, the possibility of parental, teacher or police harassment is extremely high. I also think that the physical risks associated with smoking it regularly are underestimated.

HOW SHOULD PARENTS COPE WITH BRINGING CHILDREN UP IN A DRUG-TAKING CULTURE?

Parents should give children the honest facts without distortion. Young people have inherent good sense which parents need to trust and accept. Young people may be inexperienced but they are not irrational. Parents should be able to admit to their children how they feel about drugs, but this needs to be part of a broader appreciation of what the children are going through at the time, and how they relate to you, as their parents. To view drugs in isolation is quite wrong and if young people are going to run into a problem with drugs, it is very unlikely that this is the only problem they will be experiencing. The idea that a child could be heavily into drugs and not manifest other worrying signs is highly unlikely. Heavy drug use is much more often a symptom, rather than the cause, of a disturbed personality or disrupted life-style.

The Americans have invented a powder you can scatter around that changes colour if it comes into contact with cannabis. It is said that parents in the States are buying this kit in their thousands, but the idea that parents are spying on their children in that way is abhorrent.

But what we should not overlook, and this is something I worry about with my own children, is that even the experimenter with drugs (and glue sniffing is an example of this) is in a situation of immediate risk. The risk may be small but it is real. You might well say, 'Riding a bicycle carries a risk,' and I do worry about that as well, and of course taking chances is part of growing up. My job as a parent is to minimize this by giving the best advice I can.

WHAT ABOUT THE FUTURE?

The future is very difficult to predict. The unarguable starting point is that drugs are a genuinely increasing issue today—in both availability and consumption. At the hard end of the market, the real price on the street of heroin and cocaine has gone down and their availability has gone up compared with ten years ago. Therefore the so-called 'war on drugs' is a failure.

The government's way of working is a combination of three elements: the suppression of supply, education and prevention, and treatment. All are important, but there is an over-emphasis on suppression of supply because politically this looks good. When you suppress supply you are replacing internal restraint (as encouraged with legal drugs) with external restraint—both intuitively and historically less effective. If you remove illegality from the drug scene, which, of course, carries huge risks, you make it possible to reintroduce internal restraint. But any move in that direction would involve a long period when things got worse before they got better, and this will always be seized on by the anti-legalization lobby.

Nevertheless, the existing legal policy has failed and therefore the law does need a drastic overhaul. That doesn't necessarily mean going down the route taken in the Netherlands to decriminalize drugs. Holland is said to have the highest murder rate in the world now and the hard drug scene is booming. But all life carries risk and we have to decide whether internal control by individuals or external control by the law will, in the long run, benefit more people more of the time.

Unfortunately, the decriminalization debate is dominated on both sides by people with vested interests and hidden agendas. The starting point has to be that recreational drugs are here to stay, and that the Misuse of Drugs Act requires urgent re-examination. People must find it extraordinary that doctors can prescribe heroin or amphetamines but not cannabis under any circumstances.

It does appear that things are likely to get worse, at least as long as there is a growing divide between the middle-class 'haves' and the unemployed and the dispossessed 'have nots'. Furthermore, the present system, under which it is the police at the arresting point who make decisions over whether or not to proceed, could arguably be seen as the worst of all worlds. Those who fit into a certain 'acceptable' social picture get away with a caution or less. Those who look a bit unusual, or belong to a section of the community held in lower esteem, get busted.

From my perspective of seeing the worst end of the drug scene, there is a sense that many people are irrevocably cut off from a route back into a mainstream way of life. If it is difficult as an Oxford graduate to get a job, then it is a thousand times more difficult if you are heroin or cocaine dependent and living on benefit. It would take a super-human effort to break out of that one.

We also have to accept that the majority of crime seems to be drug related. And there is the problem of the huge profits being made out of drugs. In the big cities, it is not uncommon to see 17-year-olds with a mobile phone and a Porsche, and they are not earning these on the Stock Exchange. The profits possible are beyond the wildest dreams of most people, which means that the risks criminals are willing to take constantly increase.

There are no quick fixes. As I say, drugs are here to stay. They are going to cause some people's health to deteriorate, and others are going to die. Unless we start thinking about the problem in a much more radical way, the future is bleak.

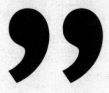

Further reading

*The Big Blue Book of Booze, In the Zone, The Lads Go Mad in
    Amsterdam, Everything You Wanted to Know about
    Cannabis, Amphetamine, MDA Snowballs*
    and many other brilliant Peanut Pete productions
    from Lifeline Manchester, 101–103 Oldham Street,
    Manchester M4 1LW. Telephone: 0161 839 2054.
    THESE ARE RATED VERY HIGHLY BY YOUNG PEOPLE
    THEMSELVES.

'Cocaine and Crack',
    and other leaflets from the Institute for the Study of
    Drug Dependency, Waterbridge House, 32–36 Loman
    Street, London SE1 0EE. Telephone: 0171 928 1211.

Drugs Problems: Where to Get Help
    and a bi-monthly newsletter, from the Standing
    Conference on Drug Abuse (SCODA), Waterbridge
    House, 32–36 Loman Street, London SE1 0EE.
    Telephone: 0171 928 9500.

*Drugs and Solvents: Things You Should Know—the Facts For Young
    People* and
    Drugs: A Parents' Guide—the Dangers: What To Do,
    both from BAPS, Health Publications Unit, DSS
    Distribution Centre, Heywood Stores, Manchester Rd,
    Heywood, Lancashire OL10 2PZ.
    Free telephone: 0800 555 777.

'Drugs: Who Takes Them, Why We Use Them, What the
Future Holds',
from *Life*, The Observer Magazine, 9, 16 and 23
October 1994.

*Forbidden Drugs: Understanding Drugs and Why People Take
Them*, by Philip Robson. Oxford Medical Publications,
1994. A WELL-REVIEWED BOOK ON THE SUBJECT OF
DRUGS.

'Roots of Addiction', *New Scientist*, 1 October 1994.

*Tackling Drugs Together: A Consultation Document on a Strategy
for England 1995–1998*

*Taking Drugs Seriously: a Parents' Guide to Young People's Drug
Use*, by Julian Cohen and James Kay. Thorsons, 1994.

'Young People and Drug-Taking: Facts and Trends',
by John Balding. *Education and Health*, Vol. 12, No. 4,
1994. THE BEST SUMMARY OF THE RATE OF DRUG
TAKING IN YOUNG PEOPLE IN THE UK.

Lamont Grandquist's guide to network drug resources, as
well as many frequently asked questions and answers
can be found on the Internet location
http://www.hyperreal.com/drugs/
and downloaded by anonymous FTP from
ftp://www.hyperreal.com/drugs/

Getting help

Cocaine Anonymous
24 hours a day
> 0171 284 1123

Drinkline
National alcohol helpline
Mon.–Fri. 9.30 a.m.–11 p.m. Sat. & Sun. 6–11 p.m.
> London only 0171 332 0202
> All UK 0345 320202

24-hour dial-and-listen line
> 0500 801802

Drugs in Schools Helpline
Nationwide confidential drug information service for pupils, parents and teachers
Mon–Fri. 10 a.m. to 5 p.m.
> 0345 366666

Family and Friends of Drug Users
Nationwide phone counselling service
> 01926 887414

Institute for the Study of Drug Dependence
Excellent source of information
> 0171 928 1211

Narcotics Anonymous
Network of self-help groups
10 a.m.–10 p.m. most days
0171 730 0009

National Drugs Helpline
Free, confidential, 24 hours a day
0800 776600

Release
Specializes in legal issues about drugs
0171 729 9904
Outside office hours
0171 603 8654

Re-Solv
Solvent abuse
Mon.–Fri. 9 a.m.–5 p.m.
01785 817885

Index

Note: **bold** page numbers indicate major entries